Prepping For Life; Macro-based, Balanced Nutrition Recipes; Volume One
First Edition
by Brandy Flotten
Published by KK Wellness Consulting, LLC

© 2018 KK Wellness Consulting, LLC

ISBN: 978-0-578-43504-6 (Paperback)

All rights reserved. No portion of this book may be reproduced in any form without permission from the publisher, except as permitted by U.S. copyright law. For permissions contact: www.kkwellnessconsulting.com

The prepping for life tagline is a registered trademark of KK Wellness Consulting, LLC

Cover by Brandy Flotten

www.kkwellnessconsulting.com

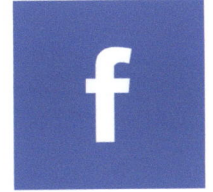  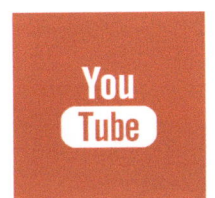 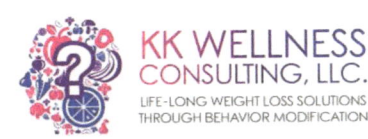

Search for us on social media; our tagline is:
#preppingforlife

Breakfast

Spinach Feta Egg White Muffins …………..……..3
Instant Pot (IP) Egg White Bites……………….....4
Cottage Cheese Waffle……………..…….....…5
Chocolate Protein Granola……………….……6
Baked Pumpkin Oatmeal ……………….…......7

Soups, Stews and Sauces

Ginger, Kale and Ground Turkey Broth……................8
Instant Pot Spaghetti Squash and Meat Sauce …....…9
Cilantro, Lime and Jalapeño Dressing …………...10

Snacks & Sides

Instant Pot Cold Start Greek Yogurt ………………11
Pizza Cottage Cheese Waffle ……………….…..12
Cocoa Egg White Muffins …………………….13
Chocolate Pumpkin Oat Protein Bars…………........14
Sweet and Spicy Sweet Potatoes………………..15
Spicy Andean Sweet Potato Dish………………...16
Cilantro Vinaigrette Sweet Potatoes …………….17
Summer Mixed Bean Salad……..………………. 18
Cumin Lime Black Bean Quinoa Salad ……………. 19
Summer Quinoa Salad…………………….…....20

Family Dinners

Instant Pot Basic Chicken…………………….....21
Flank Steak with Avocado Chimichurri Sauce……….22
Chicken Kebabs with Tzatziki Sauce ………..…….23
Greek Marinated Pork Tenderloin…………….……24
Latin Chicken and Black Bean Salad ……………...25
Buffalo Chicken Casserole…..…………………….26
Apricot Glazed Pork Tenderloin …………….…..27
Turkey Meatloaf Muffins…………………………28
Grilled Salmon with Orange Ginger Mustard Glaze ..29
Shrimp and Scallop Stir Fry……………….……...30
Crab Cakes ………………...………….…..…..31
Spicy Tuna Poke Bowls…..………………….…32

Healthy Treats

Coconut Peanut Butter Protein Balls ……………..33
Energy Balls……………………………….…..34
Black Cherry Protein Smoothie Bowl……………...35
Lemon Chickpea Muffins ……………………...…36

Spinach Feta Egg White Muffins

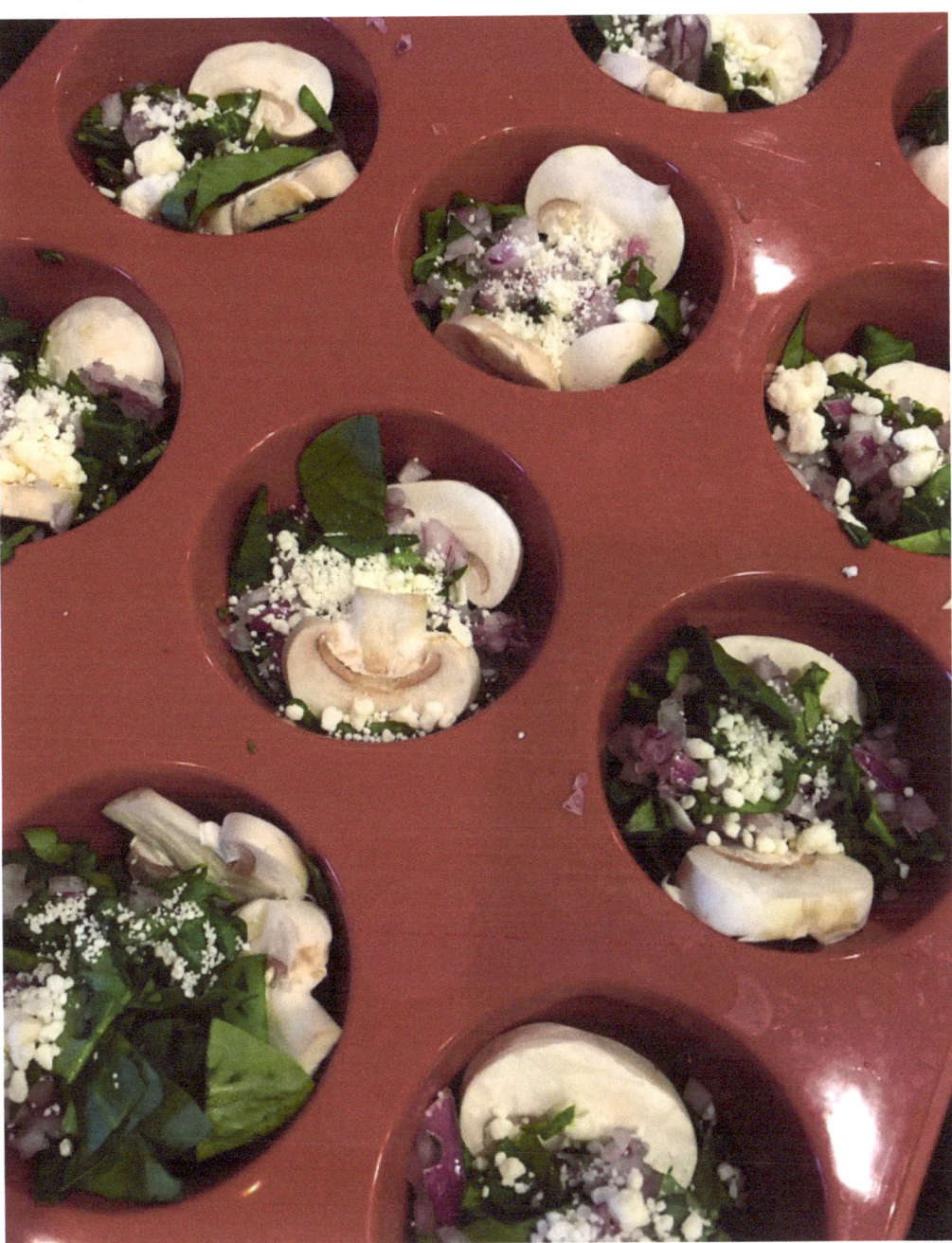

Ingredients:
32 oz. liquid egg whites
¼ cup mushroom, chopped
¼ cup red onion, chopped
1 ½ cups spinach, raw
3 Tbsp crumbled feta cheese

Variations: (macros would need to be recalculated)
turkey breakfast sausage
bacon
cheese

Yield: 12 Egg Muffins

Suggested Serving Size: 2-3 Egg Muffins

Directions:
1. Spray silicone molds or standard muffin tin with cooking spray.
2. Place silicone mold on cookie sheet before adding ingredients.
3. Add veggies evenly into muffin cavities.
4. Add ¼ tsp crumbled feta cheese into each cavity.
5. Fill each cavity to the top with liquid egg whites.
6. Bake at 325°F for 35 minutes or until eggs are done and slightly browned at edges.

Calories per serving: 51
Carbohydrates 1g, Protein 8g, Fat 1g

Instant Pot (IP) Egg White Bites

Ingredients:
14 oz. liquid egg whites
¼ cup red bell pepper, chopped
¼ cup red onion, chopped
½ cup spinach, raw
1 cup water

Variations: (macros would need to be recalculated)
feta cheese
mushrooms
breakfast meat

Yield: 7 Egg White Bites
Suggested Serving: 1-4

Directions:
1. Double recipe if using two baby food silicone molds.
2. Spray silicone molds with cooking spray.
3. Add veggies into silicone mold cavities.
4. Pour 1 cup water into Instant Pot.
5. Fill each cavity to top with liquid egg whites. Each tray uses approximately 14 oz. egg whites.
6. Carefully Stack Molds on top of trivet (rotating second mold slightly so they stack) and place in Instant Pot.
7. Close lid and venting knob. Select Manual for 9 minutes. Allow Instant Pot to natural release (approximately 12-15 minutes after cook time).
8. Open lid and remove egg white bites.

Calories: 29
Carbohydrates: 1g, Protein 5g, Fat 0g

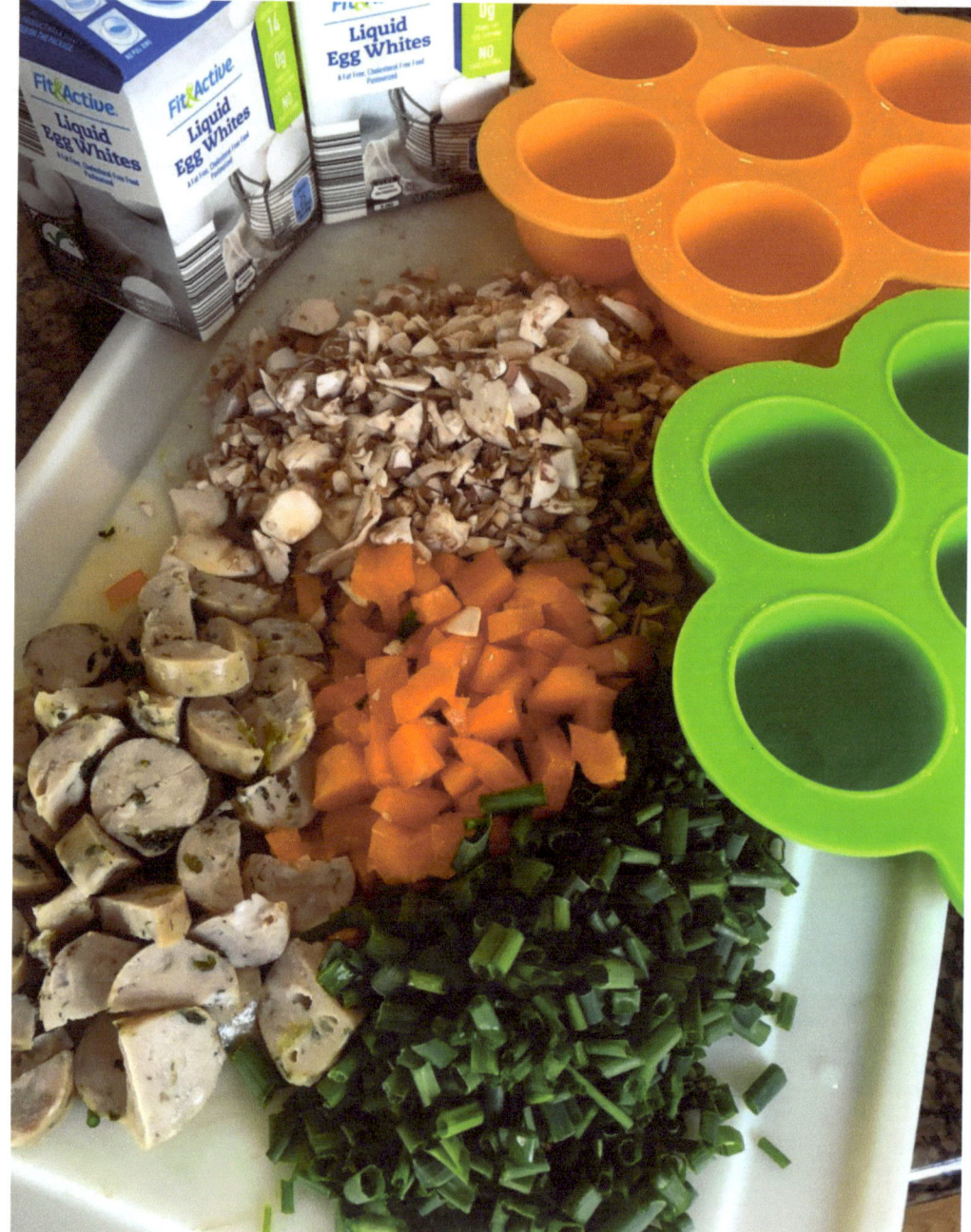

Cottage Cheese Waffle

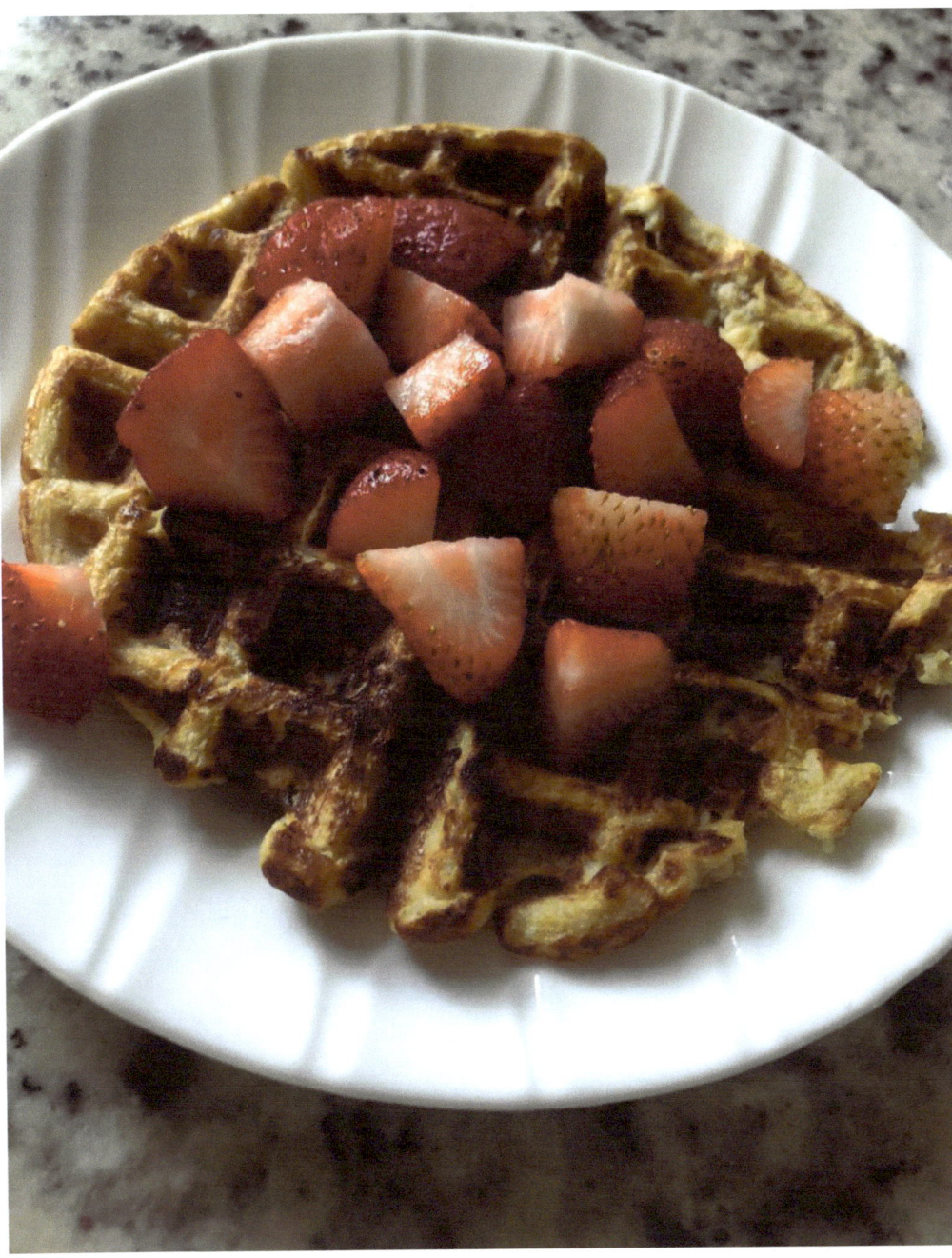

Ingredients:
1 cup Quaker oats
2 whole eggs
3 egg whites
1 cup non-fat cottage cheese
1 tsp vanilla extract
1 tsp ground cinnamon
1 tsp raw honey (optional)

Yield: 3 Waffles

Suggested Serving Size: 1 Waffle

Directions:
1. Add all ingredients in blender.
2. Blend until smooth.
3. Spray waffle iron lightly with olive oil or non-stick spray.
4. Pour in batter and cook until golden brown.
5. Enjoy!

Calories per serving: 255
Carbohydrates 24g, Protein 20g, Fat 5g

Chocolate Protein Granola

Ingredients:
5 cups Quaker rolled oats
¼ cup honey
¼ cup oil
1 cup water
1 tsp vanilla
1 tsp orange zest
½ cup pumpkin kernels, raw
1 cup (120g) of chocolate protein powder (macros will be slightly different using your protein powder)

Variations: (not calculated in macros)
unsweetened coconut
sliced almonds
dried fruit

Yield: 8 cups

Suggested Serving: ¼ cup

Directions:
1. Preheat oven to 325°F.
2. Line a large baking sheet with parchment paper.
3. Combine oats water, honey, oil, vanilla, orange zest and any optional spices in large bowl.
4. Add protein powder and mix well to evenly coat oats. Add more water if needed.
5. Mix in remaining seeds and or nuts and spread evenly on prepared baking sheet.
6. Bake for 42 to 45 minutes, stirring once or twice, or until granola is dry. Remove from oven and let cool completely on sheet. Stir in any dried fruit, if using.
7. Store cooled granola in an airtight container for up to 2 weeks, or freeze for up to 2 months.

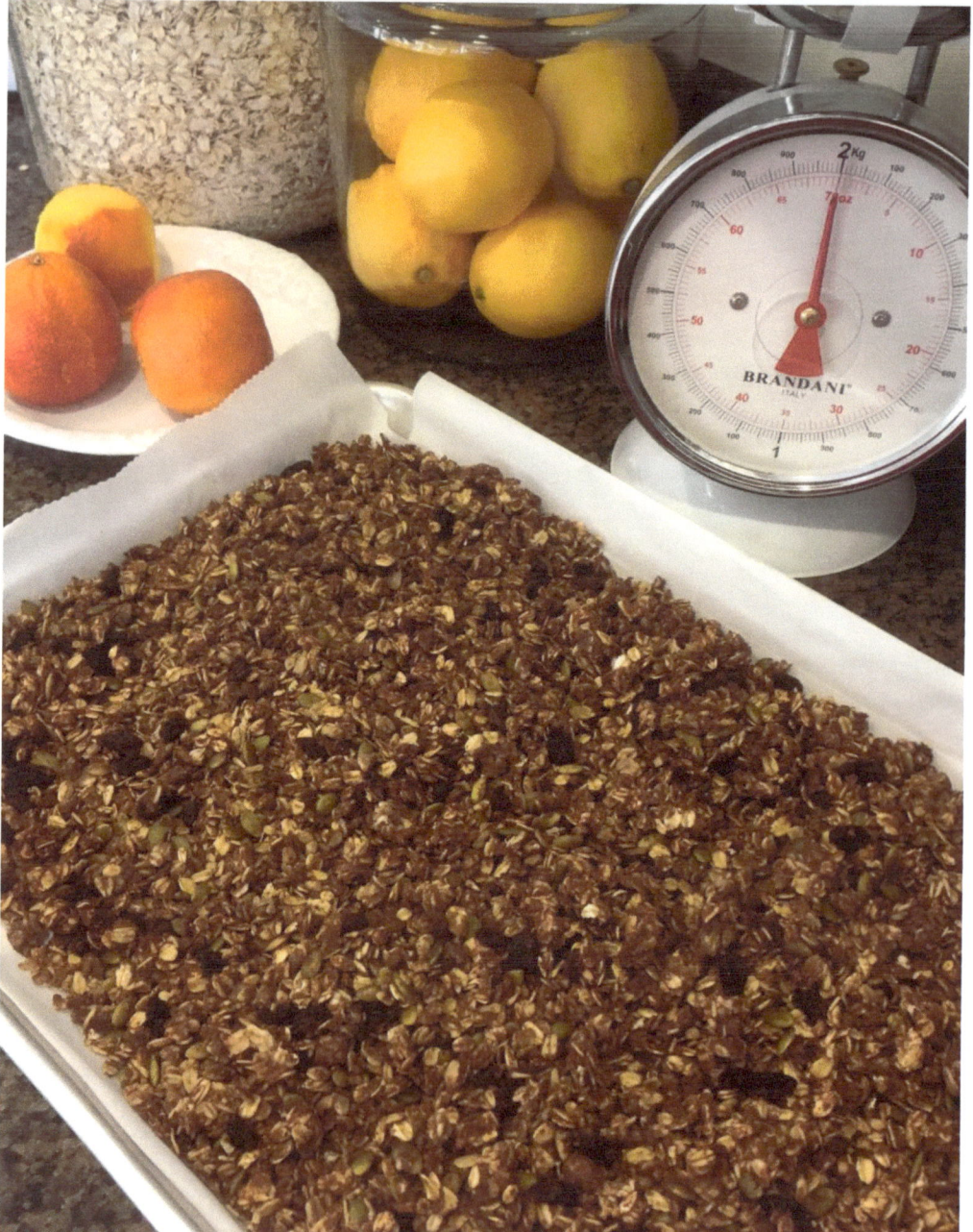

Calories per ¼ cup: 93
Carbohydrates: 12g, Protein 4g, Fat 4g

Baked Pumpkin Oatmeal

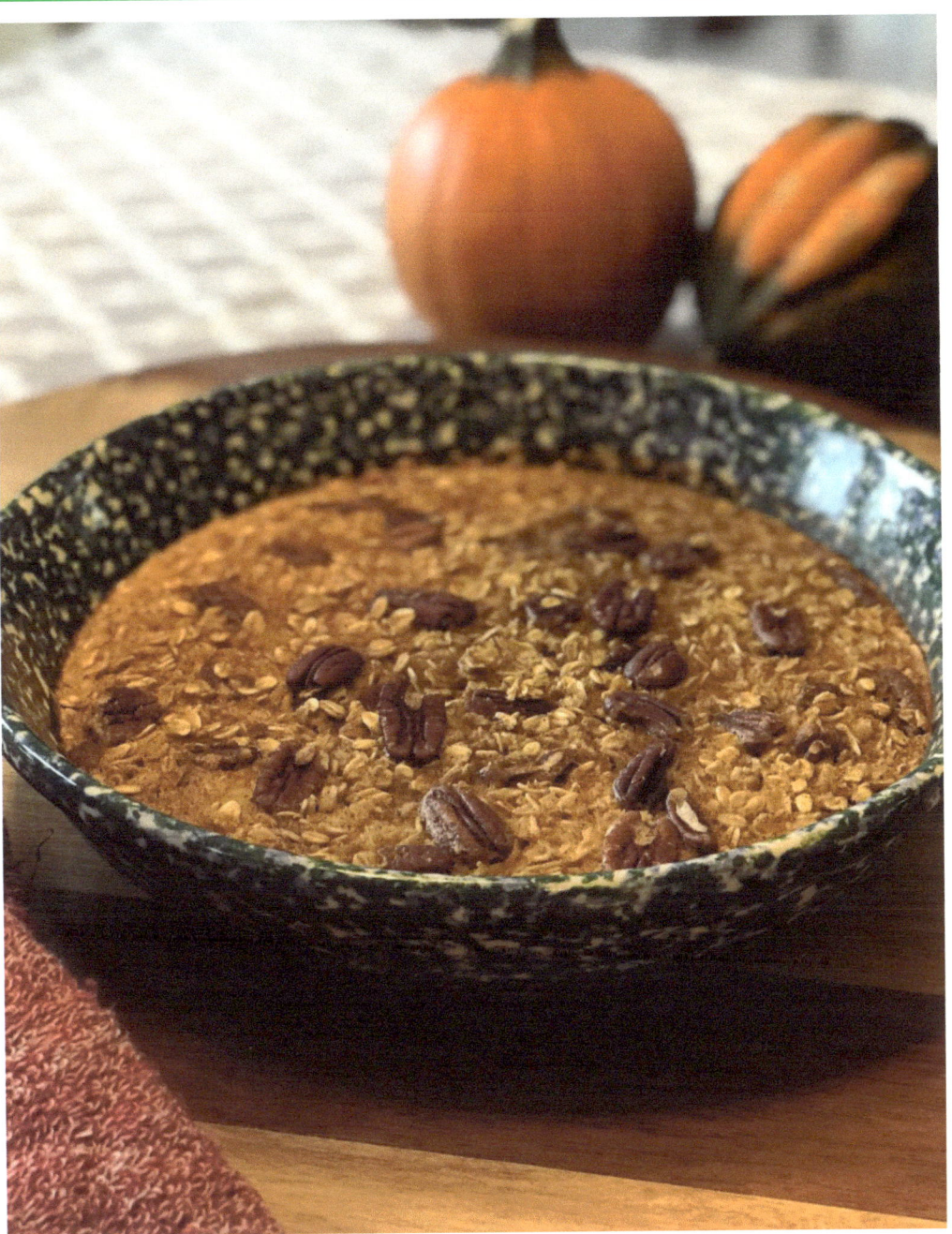

Ingredients:
- 2 cups quick oats
- ½ tsp baking powder
- ¼ tsp salt
- 1 tsp cinnamon
- ¼ tsp nutmeg
- ¼ tsp cardamom
- ½ cup pecans
- 1 ½ cups unsweetened almond milk
- 1 cup pumpkin puree
- 1 egg
- ½ tsp vanilla extract
- ¼ cup pure maple syrup (optional)

Yield: 8 Servings

Directions:
1. Preheat the oven to 350°F.
2. In a large bowl, combine all dry ingredients including pecans (reserve a few to sprinkle on top).
3. In a separate bowl, whisk together the wet ingredients: milk, pumpkin, syrup, egg, and vanilla.
4. Stir the wet ingredients into the dry oatmeal mixture until thoroughly mixed.
5. Pour into a greased 8"x8" baking dish. Sprinkle with additional pecans if desired.
6. Bake at 350°F for 25-30 minutes, or until the liquid has cooked off, the center is set, and the edges start to brown.

Calories per serving: 177
Carbohydrates 27g, Protein 4g, Fat 7g

Ginger, Kale and Ground Turkey Broth

Ingredients:
32 oz. chicken bone broth
32 oz. 99% lean ground turkey (2 packages)
1 ½ cups kale, chopped
1 ½ Tbsp grated ginger, fresh
2 Tbsp green onions
2 cups jasmine rice (not included in macros); If adding rice, add 2 cups of water

Yield: 6 Servings

(4-5 oz. Ground Turkey in each serving)

Directions:
1. Brown ground turkey in large pan.
2. Weigh ground turkey and separate into prep containers.
3. In large saucepan, combine bone broth, ginger, chopped kale, green onions, rice and water. Simmer until kale has softened and rice is cooked.
4. Add equal parts of broth mixture to your prep containers already filled with ground turkey.

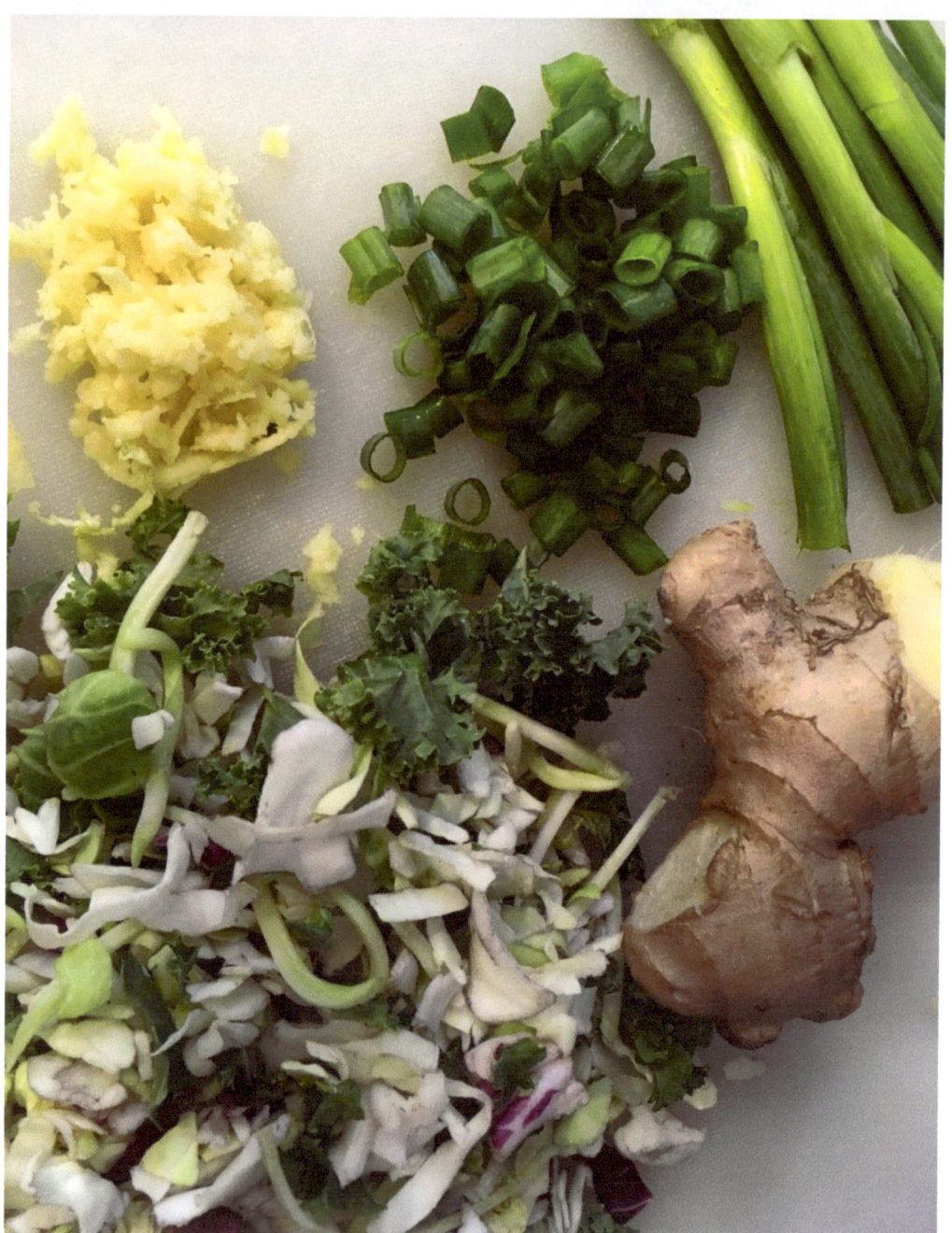

Calories: 214
Carbohydrates: 2g, Protein 43g, Fat 6g

Instant Pot Spaghetti Squash and Meat Sauce

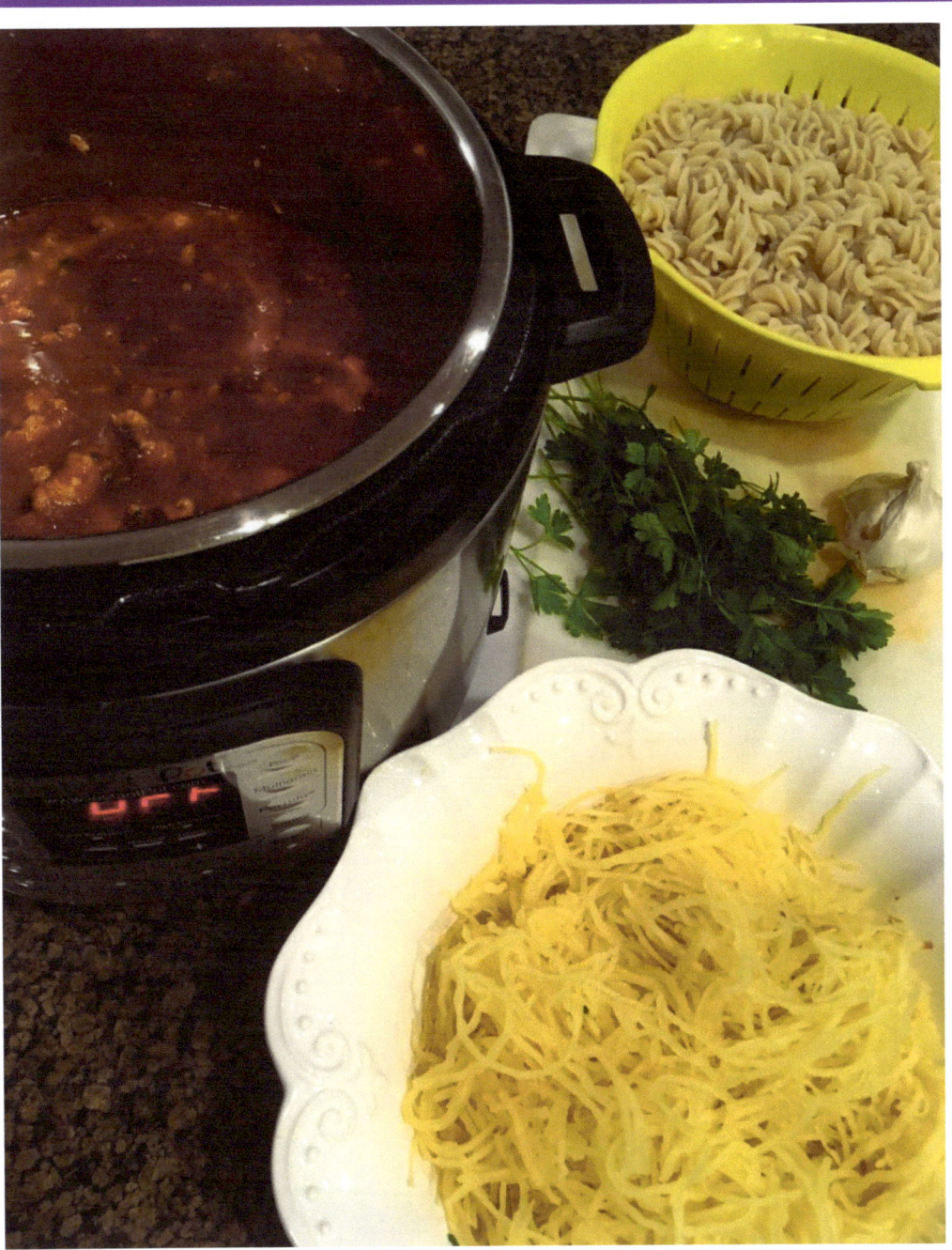

Ingredients:

16 oz. 99% lean ground turkey
16 oz. ground chicken breast
3-4 garlic cloves, minced
28 oz. diced tomatoes
6 oz. tomato paste
30 oz. tomato sauce
3 tsp basil, dried
2 tsp parsley, dried
½ tsp red pepper flakes
1 cup water
½ tsp ground black pepper
1 tsp salt (optional)
1 onion, diced (optional)
1 spaghetti squash (optional)

Yield: 6 cups
Suggested Serving Size: 1 cup Sauce

Directions:
1. Brown ground turkey and chicken in pan or in Instant Pot on sauté function. Transfer to meat to Instant Pot if browned in a pan.
2. Add the remaining ingredients to the Instant Pot.
3. Wash and pierce spaghetti squash several times and place on top of sauce in Instant Pot.
4. Close lid and venting knob. Select Manual for 10 minutes. (If your squash is large add 2-5 more minutes)
5. Allow Instant Pot to natural release (approximately 15 minutes after cook time).
6. Open lid and remove spaghetti squash. Cut in half, remove seeds and scrape from skin.
7. Serve meat sauce over spaghetti squash and/or over pasta of your choice.

Calories per cup of sauce: 288
Carbohydrates: 19g, Protein 37g, Fat 7g

Cilantro, Lime and Jalapeño Dressing

Ingredients:
- ½ cup cilantro, chopped
- 3 Tbsp almonds
- 3 Tbsp fresh squeezed lime juice
- 3 Tbsp water
- 1 garlic clove
- 1 jalapeño pepper, seeds removed
- 1 tsp cumin
- ½ tsp salt
- 2 Tbsp non-fat plain Greek yogurt

Yield: ½ cup

Suggested Serving Size: 2 Tbsp

Directions:
1. In a food processor, blend ½ cup cilantro, almonds, lime juice, water, jalapeño, garlic, cumin and salt until smooth.
2. Add greek yogurt and pulse to mix.
3. Serve on your favorite salad!

Calories per serving: 71
Carbohydrates: 3g, Protein 3g, Fat 6g

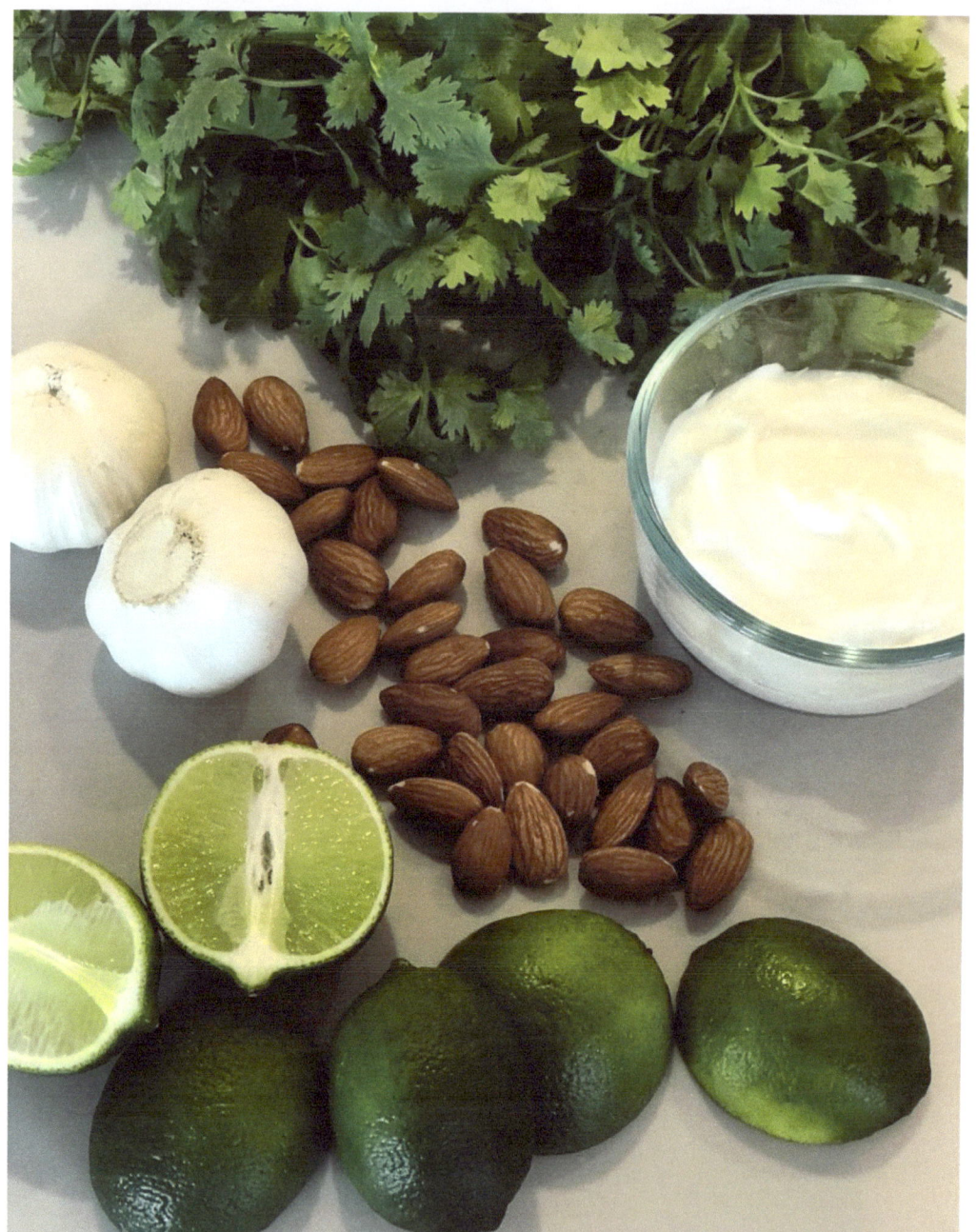

Instant Pot Cold Start Greek Yogurt

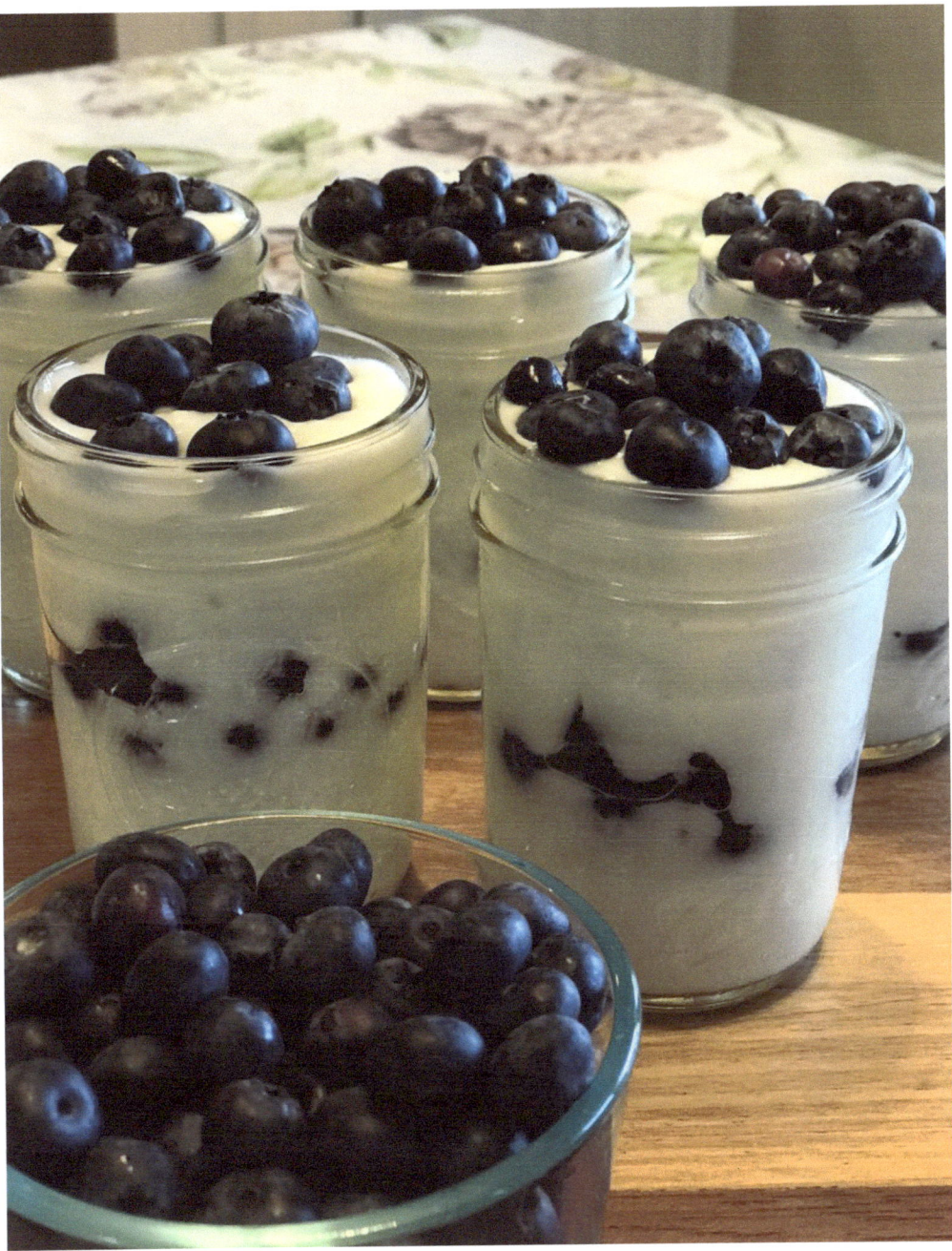

Ingredients:
1.5L fat free Fairlife milk
2 Tbsp fat-free plain Greek yogurt
1 tsp vanilla extract
1 box sugar free Jello instant pudding mix, any flavor (can be omitted)

Yield: 6 cups

Suggested Serving Size: 1 cup

Directions:
1. Mix all ingredients in Instant Pot.
2. Select "Yogurt" setting for 8 hours. If your Instant Pot does not have the pre-programmed yogurt setting, use your instruction manual to program the slow cooker setting for 180°F for 8 hours.
3. Refrigerate when done.

Calories per serving: 112
Carbohydrates 11g, Protein 15.6g, Fat 0g

Pizza Cottage Cheese Waffle

Ingredients:
1 cup Quaker oats
2 eggs, whole
3 egg whites
1 cup non-fat cottage cheese
1 cup turkey sausage crumbles
½ tsp garlic powder
¼ tsp onion powder
½ tsp red pepper flakes
¼ cup parmesan cheese (optional, not included in macros)
marinara sauce for dipping

Yield: 4 Waffles

Suggested Serving Size: 1 waffle

Directions:
1. Add all ingredients in blender with the exception of the sausage crumbles.
2. Blend until smooth.
3. Add Sausage crumbles and pulse a few times.
4. Spray waffle iron lightly with olive oil or non-stick spray.
5. Pour in batter and cook until golden brown.
6. Serve with a side of marinara sauce.

Calories per waffle: 321
Carbohydrates: 45g, Protein 24g, Fat 6g

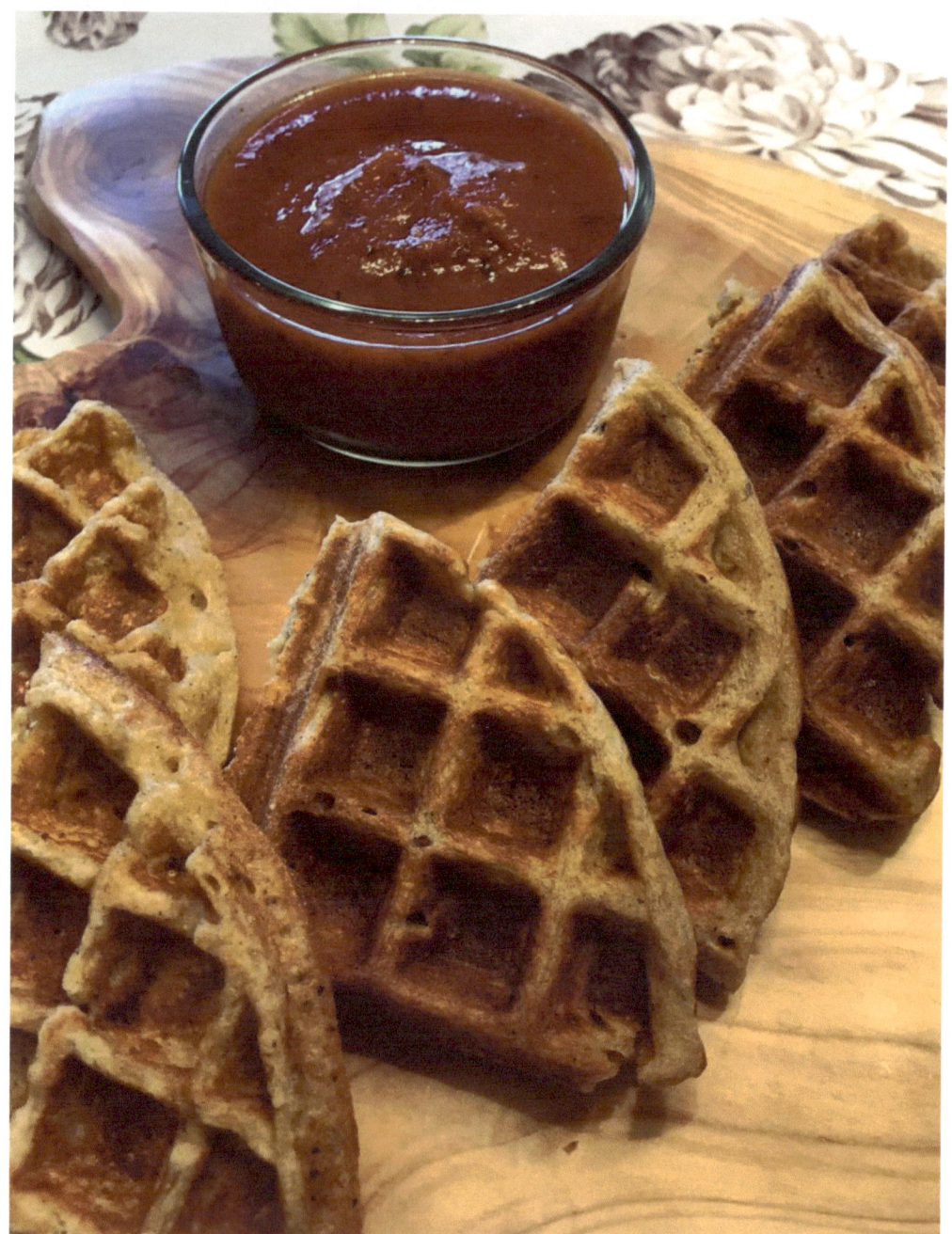

Cocoa Egg White Muffins

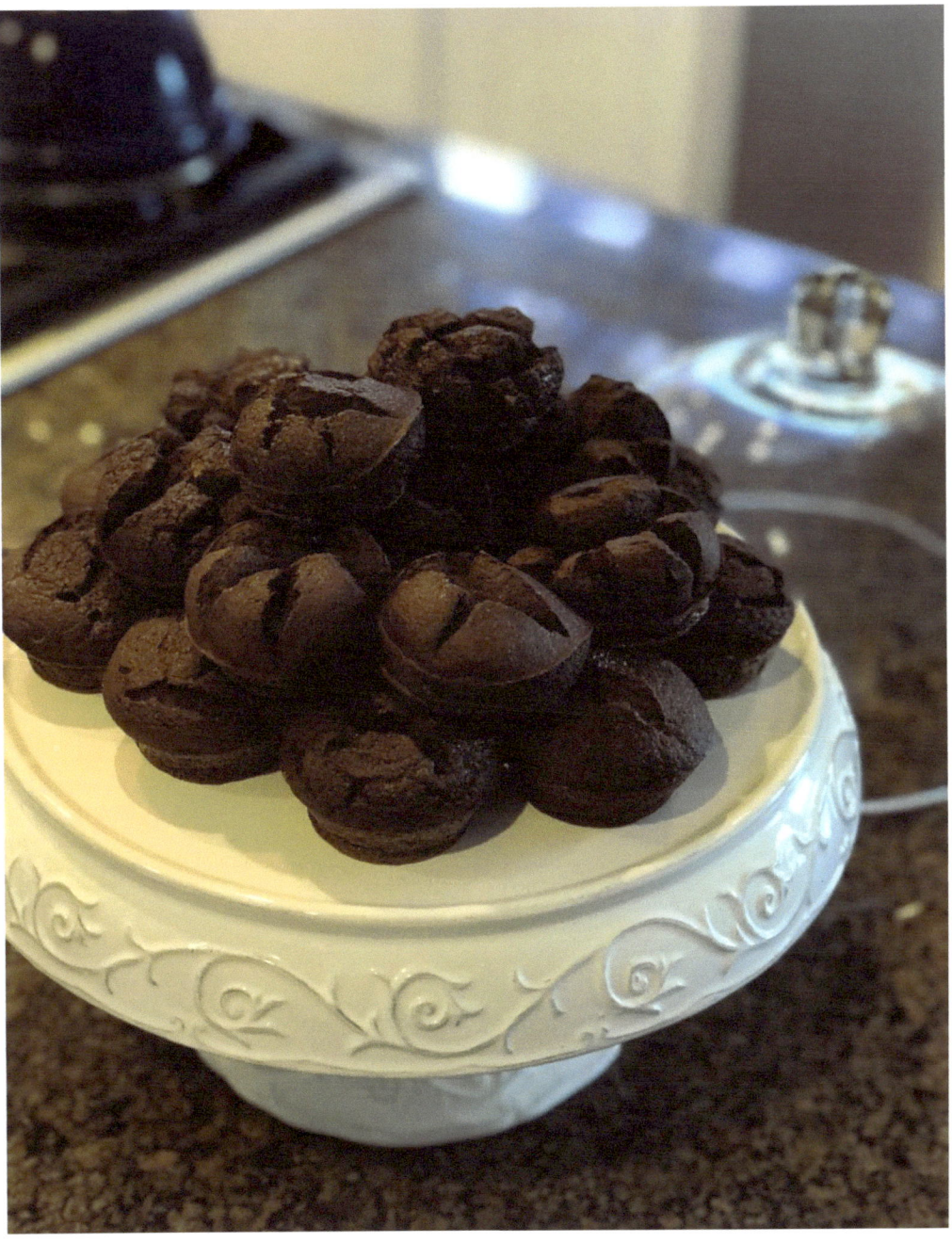

Ingredients:
4 cups liquid egg whites
2 cups Quaker oats
2 tsp baking powder
1 tsp baking soda
1 banana
4.9 oz. unsweetened applesauce
¼ cup cacao (or Hershey's dark cocoa powder)
1 tsp cinnamon
1 tsp vanilla
¼ cup Pbfit peanut butter powder
¼ -½ cup Stevia or sweetener of your choice (optional)

Yield: 18 Muffins

Directions:
1. Spray muffin pan with olive oil or baking spray. (Silicone muffin molds make clean-up much easier.)
2. Place all ingredients in blender and blend on high for 30-60 seconds.
3. Quickly pour liquid into muffin pans (so the oats don't settle to the bottom).
4. Cook for 30 minutes at 350°F or until toothpick inserted into muffin comes out clean.
5. Let cool and portion into bags of 2 or 3 (to meet your macros)
6. Store in Refrigerator or Freeze!

Calories per muffin: 79
Carbohydrates 10g, Protein 8g, Fat 1g

Chocolate Pumpkin Oat Protein Bars

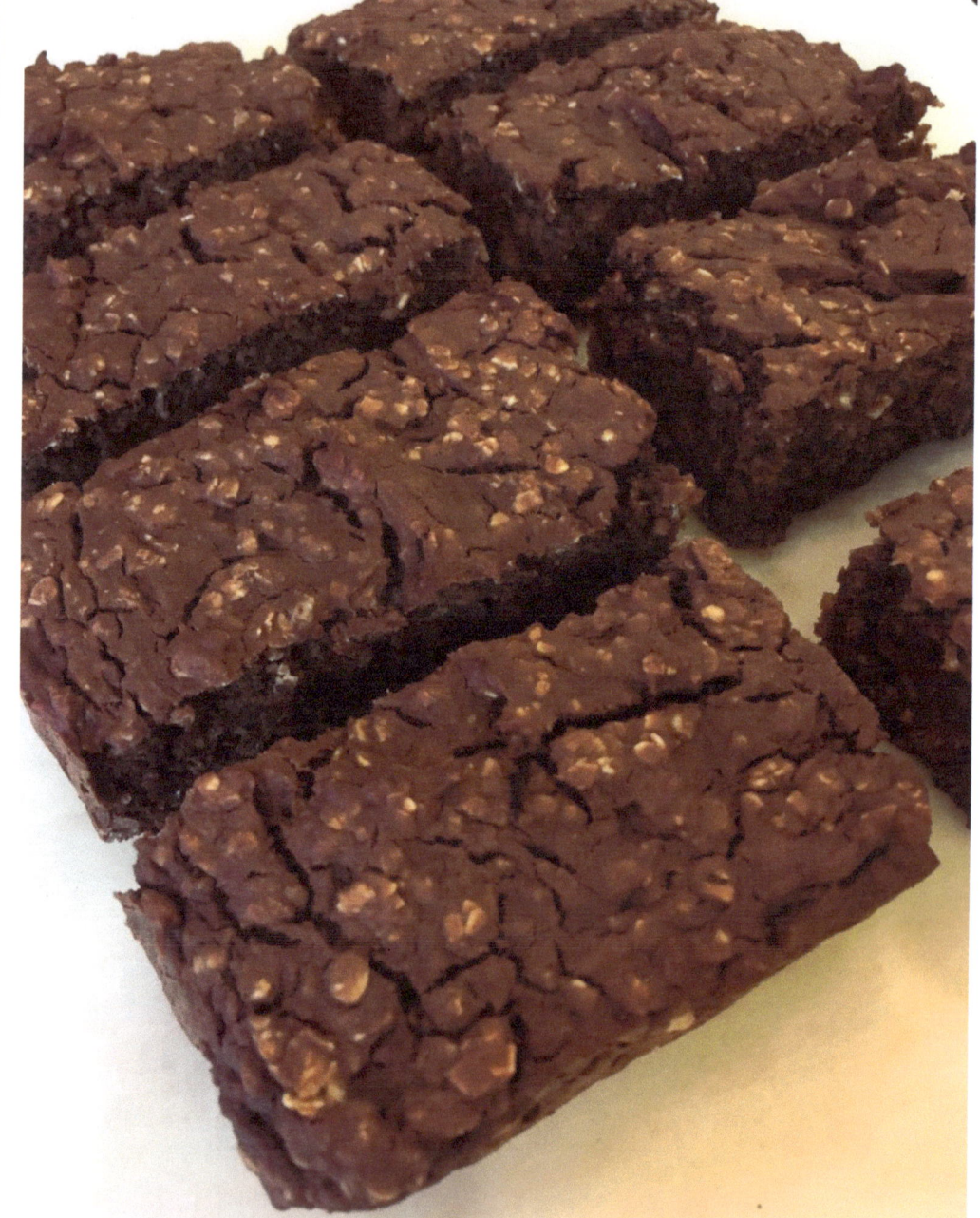

Ingredients:
1 cup pumpkin puree
1 cup applesauce, unsweetened
½ cup egg whites
¼ cup maple syrup (or baking Stevia)
1 tsp vanilla extract
2 ½ tsp pumpkin pie spice
1 tsp baking powder
½ tsp baking soda
¾ cup chocolate protein powder
1 ½ cups quick or old fashioned rolled oats
½ cup PBfit peanut butter powder (optional)

Yield: 8 bars

Directions:
1. Preheat oven to 375°F.
2. Line 8" x 8" square baking dish with parchment paper and spray with cooking spray. Set aside.
3. Whisk together pumpkin puree, applesauce, egg whites, maple syrup (or stevia), vanilla extract, pumpkin pie spice, baking powder, baking soda and PBfit and protein powder. Add oats, stir well.
4. Pour mixture in prepared baking dish, level with spatula and bake for 35 minutes or until a toothpick inserted in the center comes out clean. Remove from the oven, let cool for 10 minutes and transfer to a cooling rack to cool for another 30 minutes.
5. Cut with a serrated knife into 8 bars. Serve warm or cold.
6. Refrigerate any leftovers!

** Macros will be slightly different with your choice of protein powder.

Calories per bar: 159
Carbohydrates: 29g, Protein 12g, Fat 3g

Sweet and Spicy Sweet Potatoes

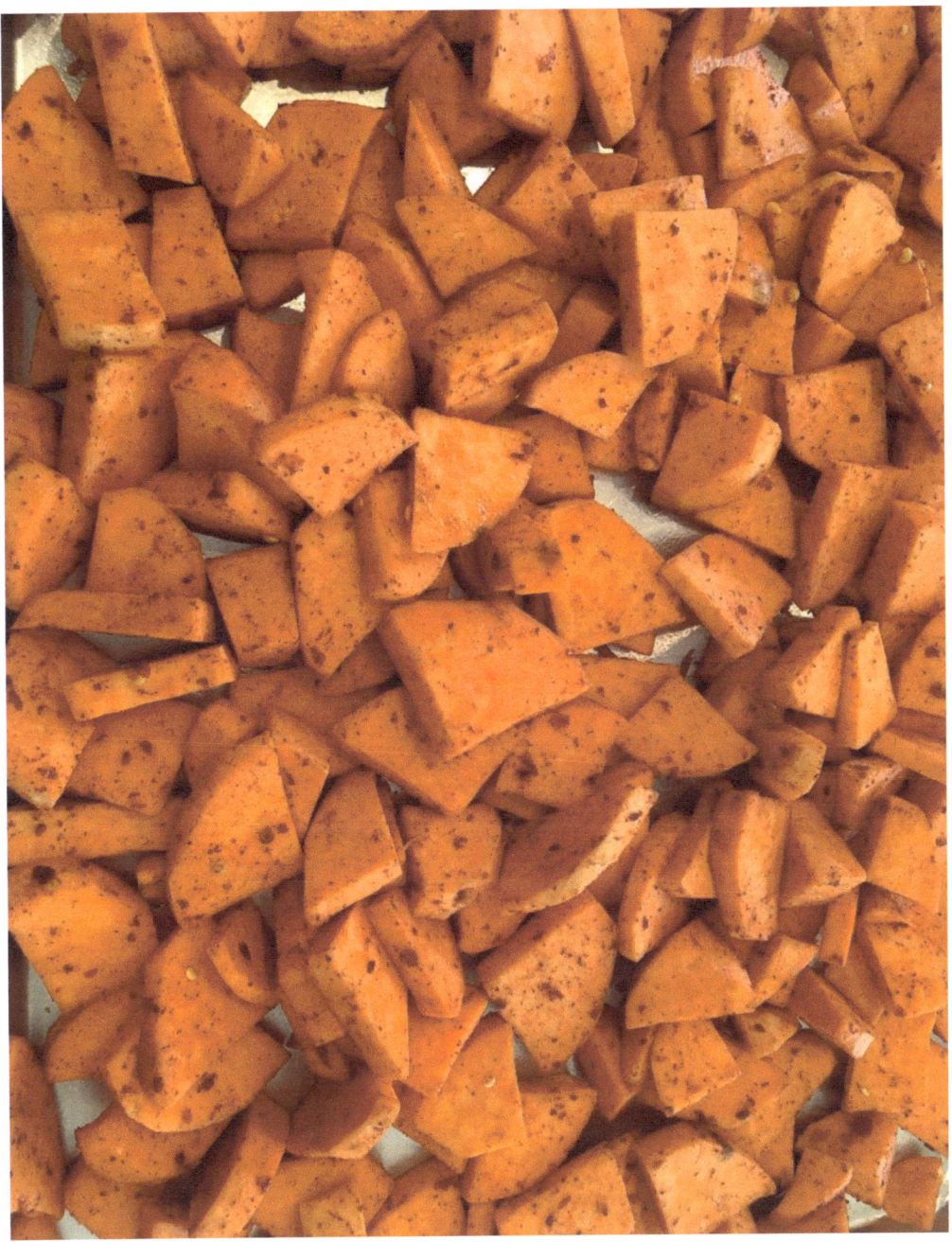

Ingredients:

4 cups sweet potatoes, peeled and cubed

2 Tbsp Sambal Oelek (ground fresh chili paste) – look for this in the grocery store next to Sriracha hot sauce!

1 ground cinnamon

1 tsp pure maple syrup (optional)

Yield: 4 cups

Suggested Serving Size: ½ cup

Directions:

1. Peel and cube sweet potatoes.
2. In a large bowl, add 2-3 Tbsp Sambal Oelek (ground fresh chili paste) and maple syrup and mix thoroughly to coat potatoes.
3. Transfer potatoes to cookie sheet and sprinkle with cinnamon.
4. Bake at 425°F for 25-30 minutes or until potatoes can be pierced easily with a fork.
5. These are great served warm or cold!

Calories per serving: 60

Carbohydrates 14g, Protein 1g, Fat 0g

Spicy Andean Sweet Potato Dish

Ingredients:
2 lbs. sweet potatoes, roasted and skins removed
1 cup sweet Vidalia onion, chopped
28 oz. crushed or diced tomatoes
1 Tbsp natural peanut butter
1 tsp cayenne pepper (optional)

Garnish:
2 tsp Parmesan cheese, grated

Yield: 8 Servings

Directions:

1. Place the potatoes in your Instant Pot with 1 cup of water. Set to manual for 18 minutes with a Natural Release. Alternatively, you can bake your potatoes in the oven at 350°F for 1 hour to get the same effect.
2. Let potatoes cool and remove skins.
3. Mash potatoes in the bottom of a small casserole dish.
4. Sprinkle cayenne pepper on top of potatoes to taste.
5. In a medium pan, sauté onions until brown. Add tomatoes and juice from can (to desired texture), peanut butter, and cayenne (to taste).
6. Stir until peanut butter is mixed in well.
7. Pour tomato sauce mixture over mashed sweet potatoes and cook at 450°F for approximately 20 minutes until hot and bubbly.
8. Garnish with freshly grated parmesan cheese and serve!

Calories: 113
Carbohydrates: 22g, Protein 4g, Fat 1g

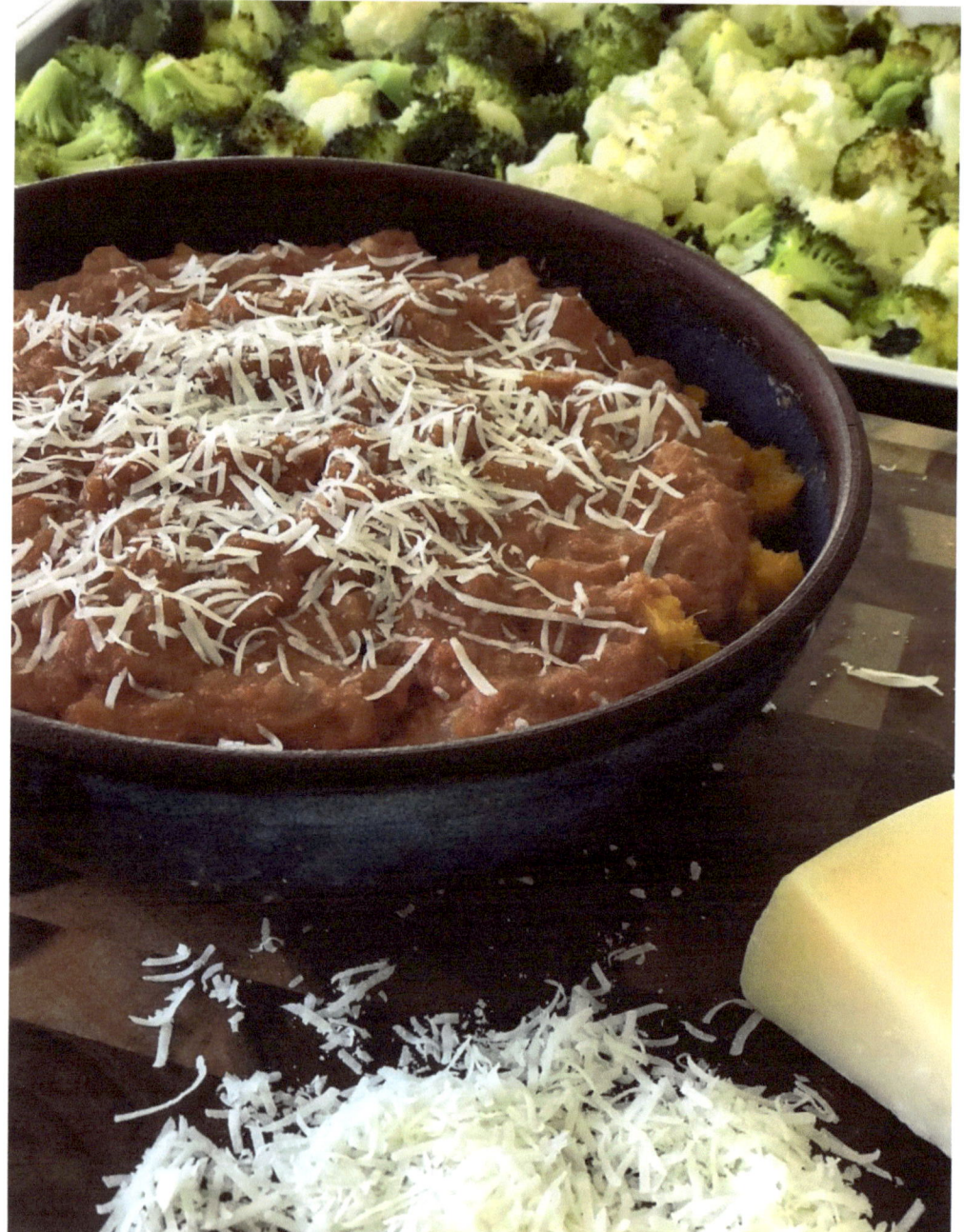

Cilantro Vinaigrette Sweet Potatoes

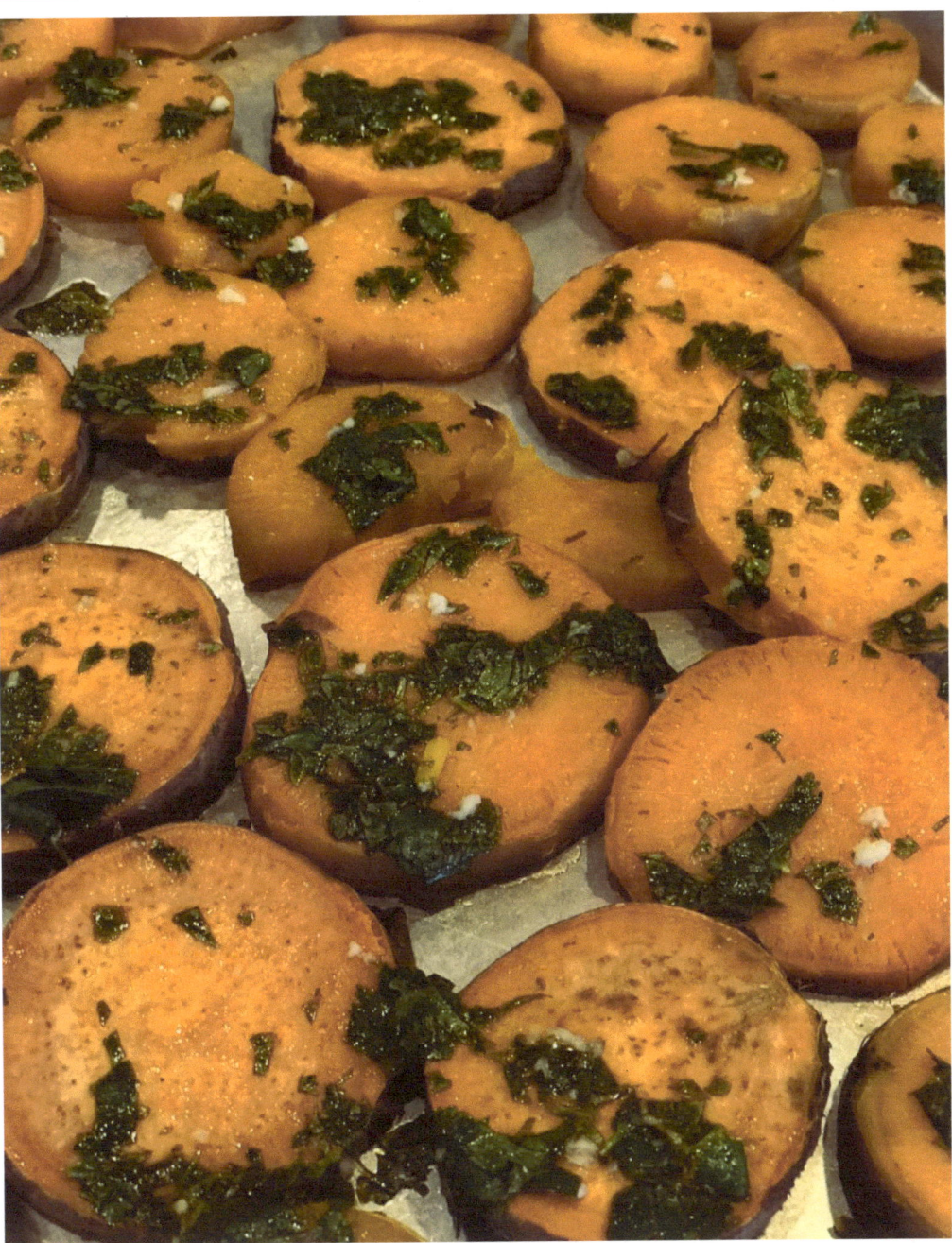

Ingredients:
3-4 sweet potatoes, sliced (approx. 24 oz)

Vinaigrette:
1 Tbsp olive oil
2 Tbsp lime juice
2 Tbsp cilantro, chopped
1 garlic clove, minced
½ tsp Agave nectar
¼ tsp salt

Yield: (6) 4oz. Servings

Directions:
1. Place the potatoes in your Instant Pot with 1 cup of water. Set to manual for 5 minutes with a Natural Release. This will pre-cook your potatoes so they are easier to slice, but still slightly firm. Alternatively, you can boil the potatoes for 20 minutes to get the same effect.
2. Slice sweet potatoes in ¼" wedges.
3. Lightly spray olive oil or cooking spray on cookie sheet and place potato wedges in a single layer.
4. Cook at 425°F for approximately 10 minutes until edges are browned.
5. Brush vinaigrette on potato wedges and serve!

Calories: 124
Carbohydrates 25g, Protein 2g, Fat 2g

Summer Mixed Bean Salad

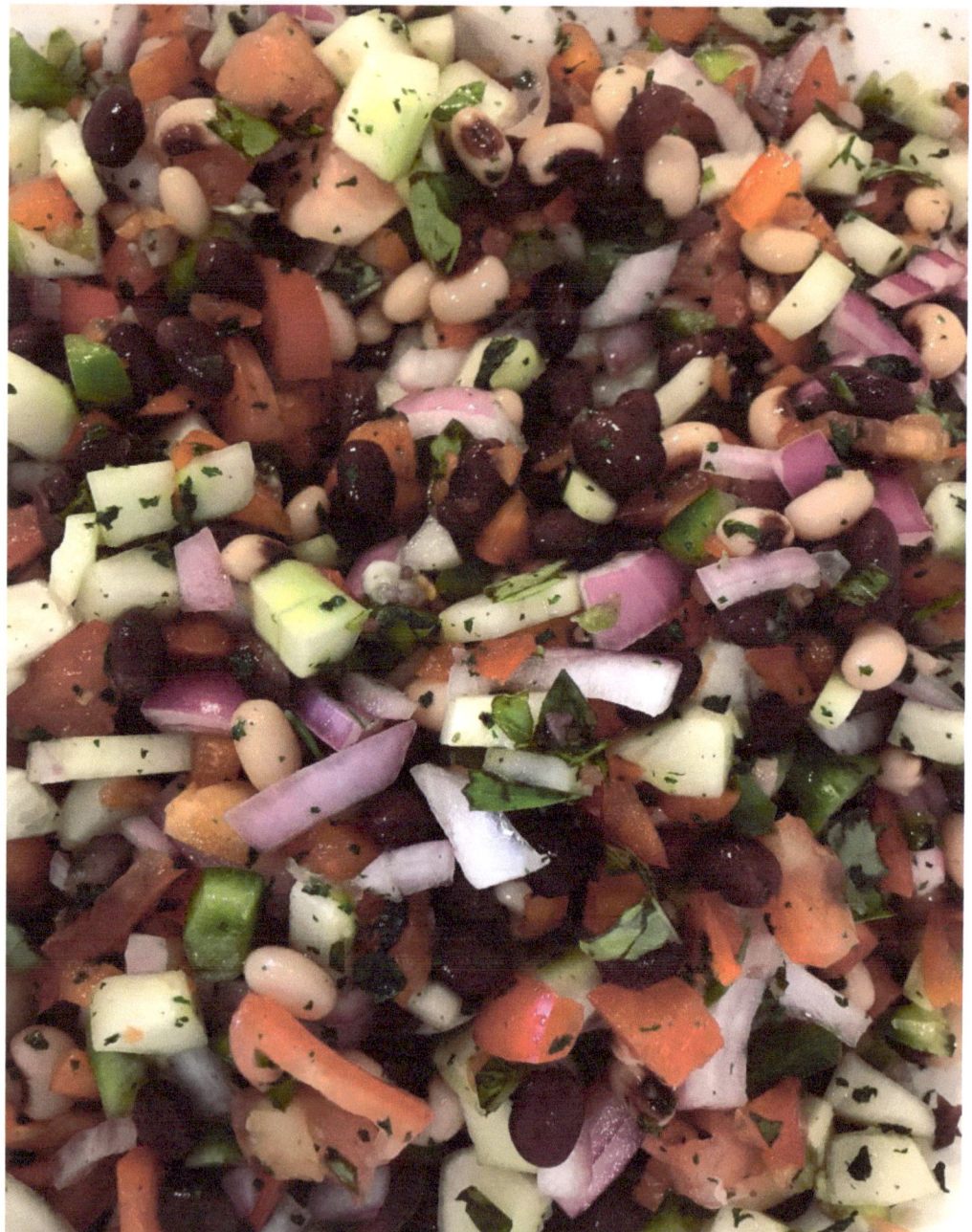

Ingredients:
(2) 15.5 oz. cans black beans
(1) 15.5 oz. can black eye peas
1 red bell pepper
½ green bell pepper
½ red onion, chopped
1 tomato (de-seeded, chopped)
juice from 1 lime
3 Tbsp red wine vinegar
½ jalapeño, finely chopped
2 cucumbers, peeled, de-seeded, and chopped
3 Tbsp fresh basil
3 Tbsp fresh mint
3 Tbsp fresh cilantro
Optional: ½ cup Feta cheese (not included in macros)

Yield: 8 cups, 16 servings

Suggested serving size: ½ cup

Directions:
1. Drain and rinse beans and peas. Pour into large bowl.
2. Peel and de-seed cucumber. Remove seeds from bell peppers, tomatoes and jalapeño. Chop all vegetables and add to the bowl.
3. Chop basil, mint and cilantro and add to the bowl.
4. Next, add juice from lime, and red wine vinegar.
5. Mix well and serve. Enjoy!

Calories: 93
Carbohydrates: 17g, Protein 5g, Fat 1g

Cumin Lime Black Bean Quinoa Salad (recipe adapted from ohsheglows.com)

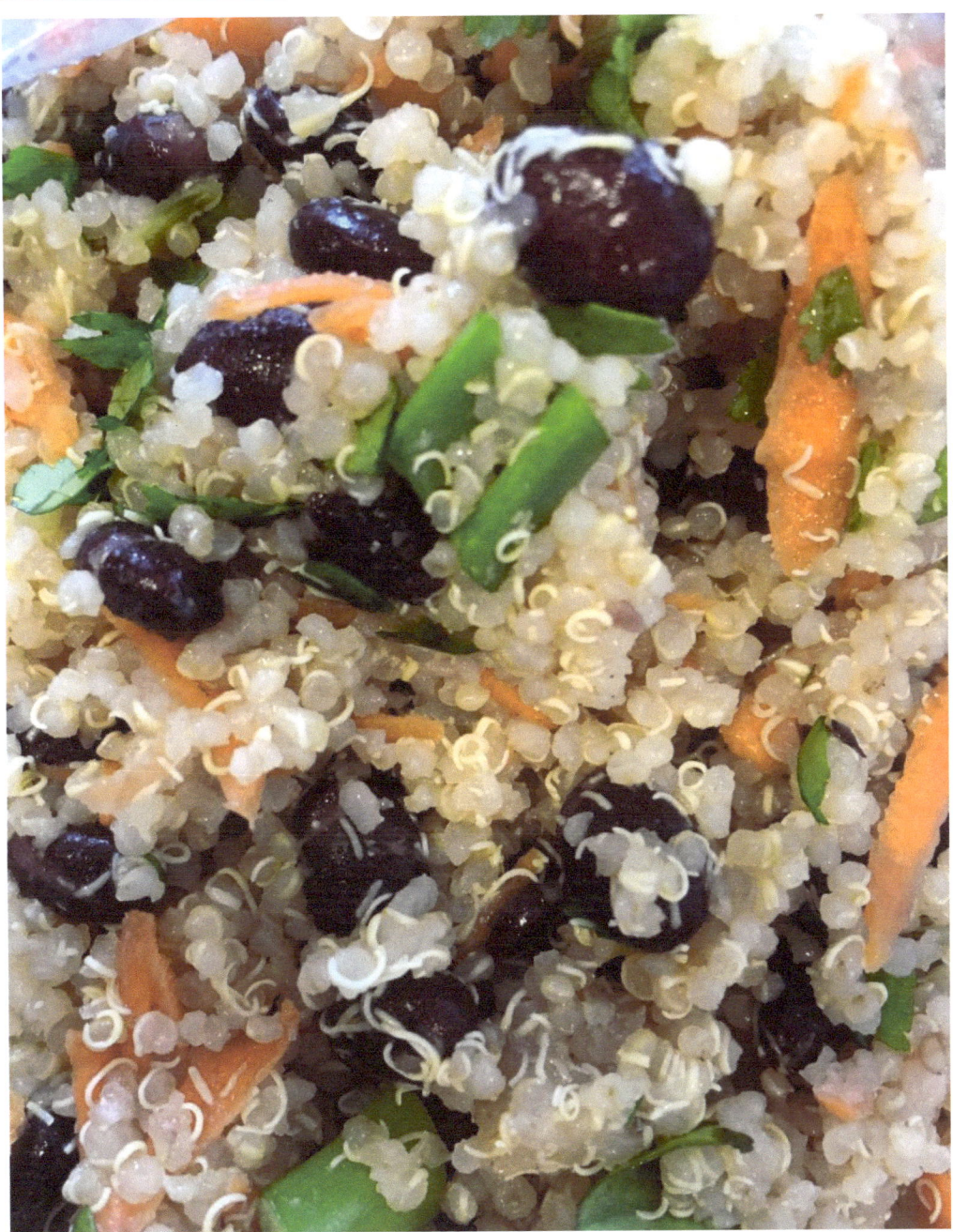

Ingredients:
1 cup quinoa (measured dry)
1 (15-oz.) can black beans
1 ½ cup fresh cilantro, chopped
1 small carrot, grated
½ cup thinly sliced green onions

Dressing:
3 Tbsp fresh lime juice
2 Tbsp extra virgin olive oil
1 tsp ground cumin
1 tsp pure maple syrup (optional)
½ tsp salt
1 garlic clove, minced

Variations:
sweet and spicy roasted sweet potatoes
prepped chicken

Yield: (6) ½ cup servings

Directions:
1. To prepare the quinoa: rinse quinoa in a fine mesh sieve.
2. Combine quinoa and 1 cup water to saucepan. Bring to a boil, reduce heat to low, and then cover with a tight-fitting lid. Simmer for 15 minutes until the water is absorbed and the quinoa is fluffy. Fluff with fork and chill in the fridge for at least 15 minutes.
3. In a large bowl, combine the quinoa, drained and rinsed black beans, cilantro, carrots and green onions. Whisk together the dressing in a small bowl or jar. Pour onto salad and toss to combine.
4. Variations: Add sweet & spicy roasted sweet potatoes and/or roasted chicken breast.

Calories per ½ cup: 228
Carbohydrates: 34g, Protein: 9g, Fat: 7g

Summer Quinoa Salad

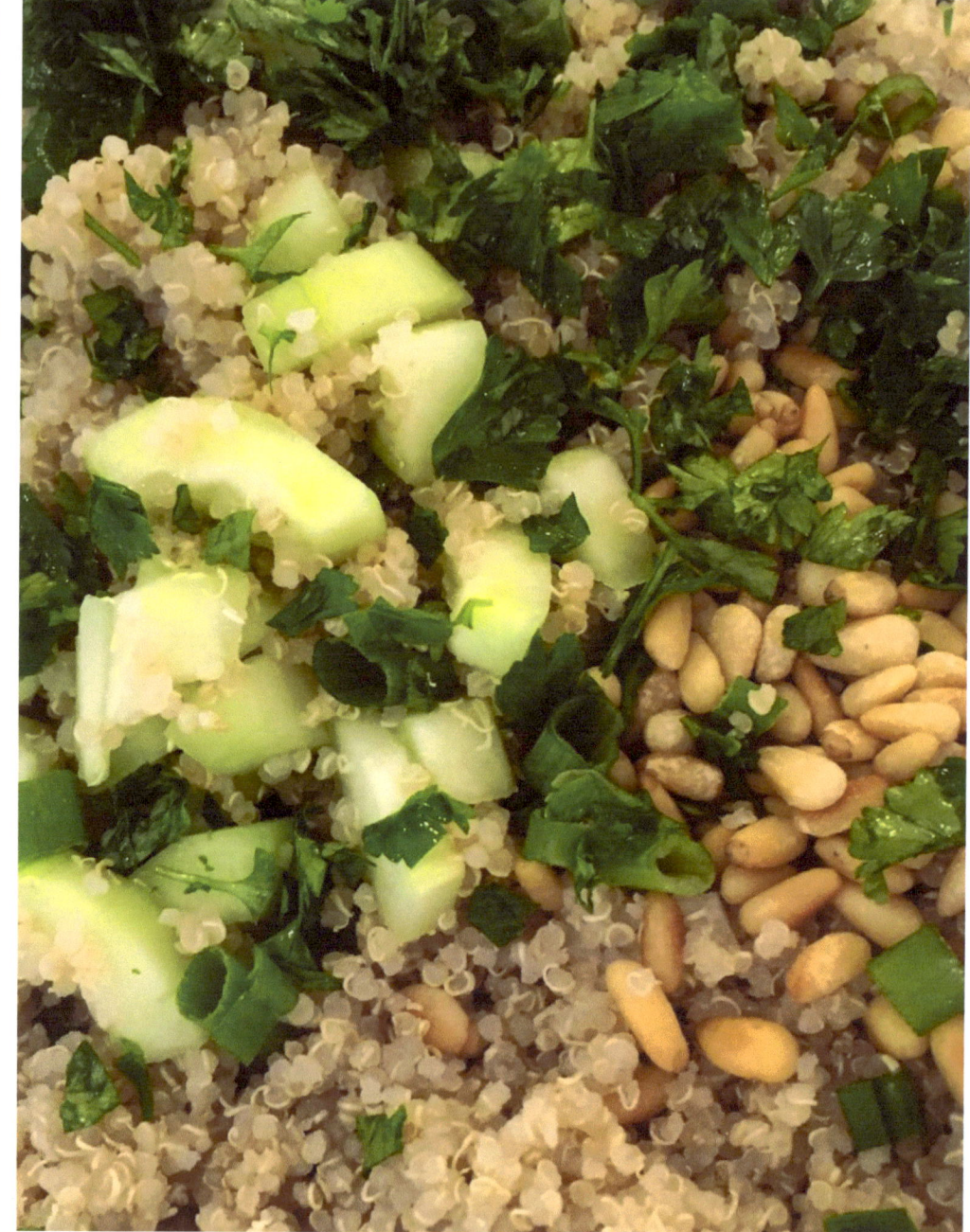

Ingredients:
1 cup quinoa (measured dry)
½ cup green onions, chopped
1 cup cucumber, peeled, seeded and chopped
¼ cup fresh flat-leaf parsley, chopped
2 Tbsp pine nuts, toasted (optional)

Dressing:
1 ½ Tbsp extra virgin olive oil
¼ cup apple cider vinegar
1 tsp ground cumin
½ tsp salt
⅛ tsp ground pepper
1 garlic clove, minced

Salad Yield: 5 cups, Dressing Yield: 3 oz.
Suggested Serving Size: ½ cup

Directions:
1. To prepare salad, follow directions on quinoa package, or you can cook it in the Instant Pot for 8 minutes on Manual.
2. Fluff quinoa with a fork. Spoon quinoa into a large bowl and cool in refrigerator. (This can be done the day before.)
3. Peel cucumbers. Slice in half and remove seeds with a spoon. Once seeds are removed, chop into small bite size pieces.
4. Add chopped green onions, cucumber, parsley and toasted pine nuts to the quinoa; toss gently to combine.
5. To prepare dressing, combine vinegar and remaining ingredients, stirring with a whisk. Drizzle dressing over salad, toss to combine.
6. Variation: Add 4 cups Cubed Prep Chicken for a 1-Dish Meal.

Calories per ½ cup serving: 90
Carbohydrates: 13g, Protein 3g, Fat 3g

Instant Pot Basic Chicken

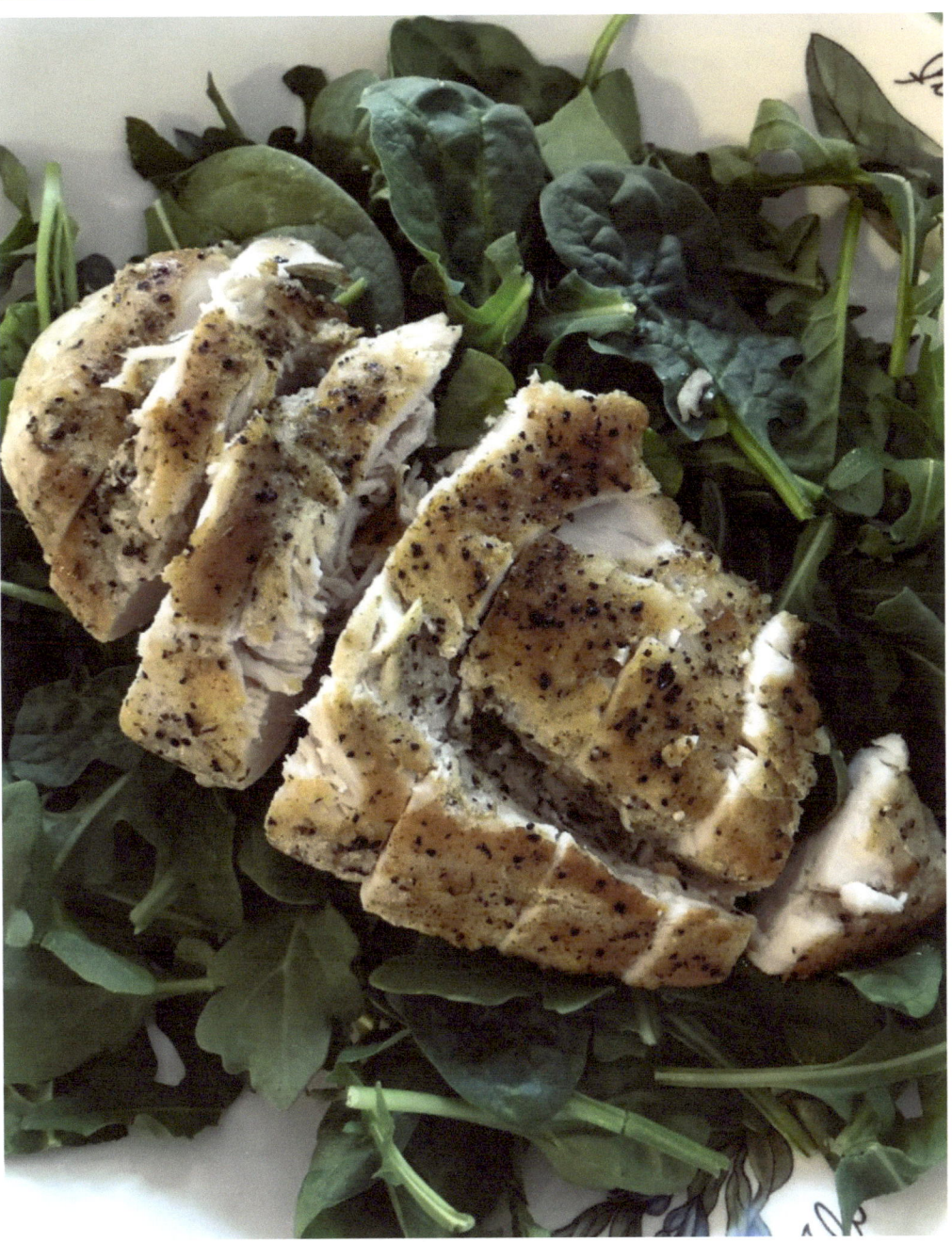

Ingredients:
4-5 Chicken Breasts
1 Tbsp Extra virgin olive oil
Seasonings of your choice

Yield: 4-5 Chicken Breasts

Directions:
1. Trim any excess fat off of chicken breasts. Season both sides with your favorite seasonings.
2. Heat 1 Tbsp extra virgin olive oil in pan.
3. Brown both sides of chicken (or you can brown your chicken breasts in the Instant Pot using the sauté function). Once browned remove, transfer chicken breasts to a plate.
4. Place trivet in Instant pot, and add 1 cup water.
5. Transfer chicken breasts to Instant Pot by laying side by side on top of the trivet.
6. Close lid and venting knob.
7. Select manual for 5 minutes.
8. Quick release pressure when done cooking.
9. Let chicken cool slightly for a few minutes. Slice and weigh chicken into appropriate portion sizes.

Calories per 5 oz. serving: 200
Carbohydrates: 0g, Protein 43g, Fat 3g

Flank Steak with Avocado Chimichurri Sauce

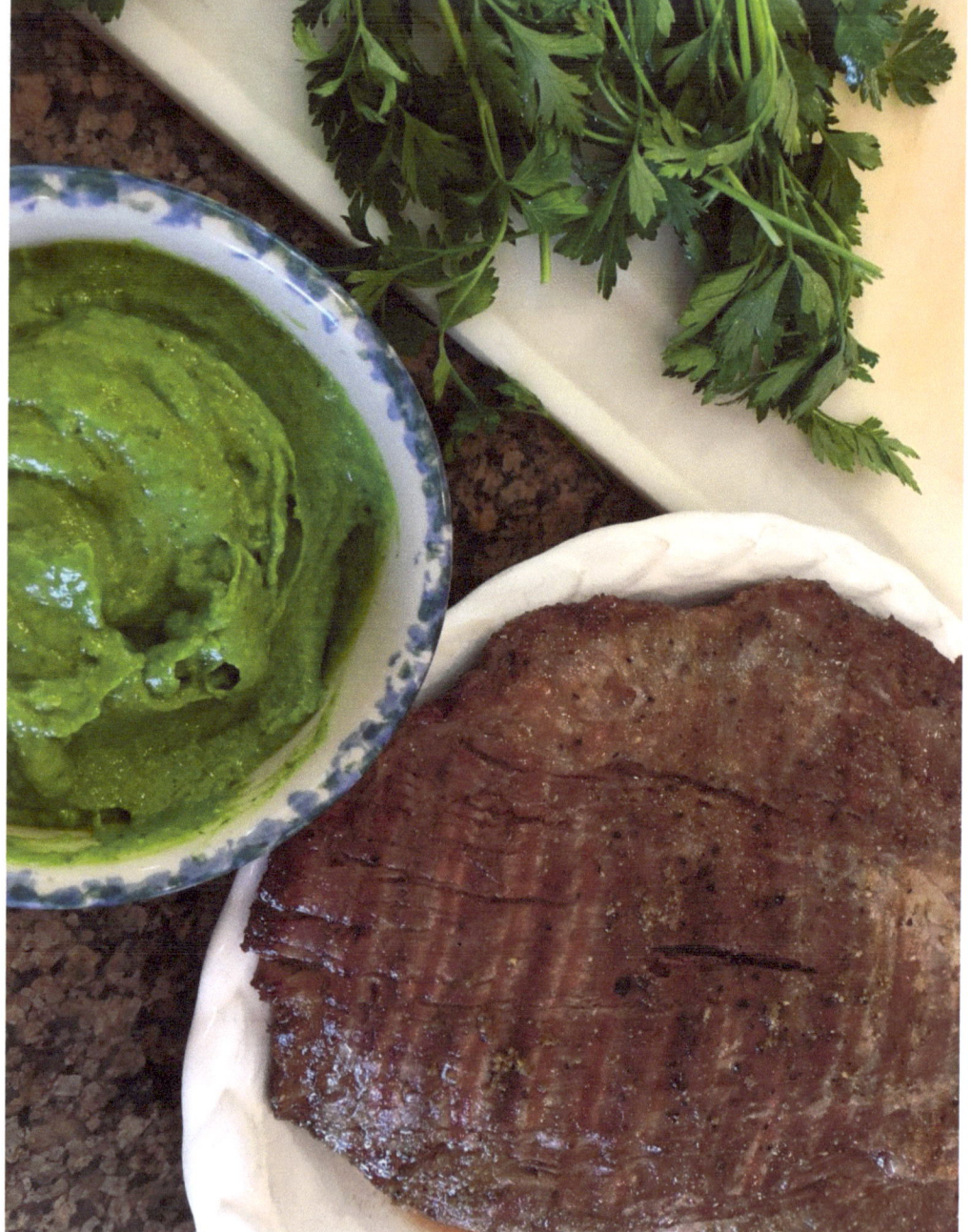

Ingredients:
1 ½-2 lbs. flank steak

Rub:
½ Tbsp ground cumin
1 tsp salt
¼ tsp ground pepper
1 Tbsp olive oil

Chimichurri Sauce:
¼ cup extra virgin olive oil
¼ cup fresh lime juice
3 cloves garlic
1 cup flat leaf parsley
½ tsp dried oregano
⅛ cayenne pepper
¼ tsp red pepper flakes
½ tsp salt
¼ tsp ground pepper
1 avocado, peeled, pitted and diced

Yield: 1 cup sauce, ~16 Servings

Recommended Serving Size; 1 Tbsp

Directions:

Steak:
1. Combine cumin, salt, and pepper in a small bowl. Rub on steak on both sides.
2. Drizzle olive oil over steak and turn to coat.
3. Preheat grill to medium-high heat.
4. Transfer steak to grill and cook until done (about 5 minutes/side for medium rare ~145°F
5. Once done, let steak rest for 5 minutes, cut in strips & serve.

Chimichurri Sauce:
1. Add oil, lime juice, garlic, parsley, oregano, cayenne pepper, red pepper flakes, salt and fresh ground pepper to a food processor or blender; pulse until herbs are finely chopped.

Chimichurri Sauce Calories/Tbsp: 25
Carbohydrates 1g, Protein 0g, Fat:2.4g

Chicken Kebabs with Tzatziki Sauce

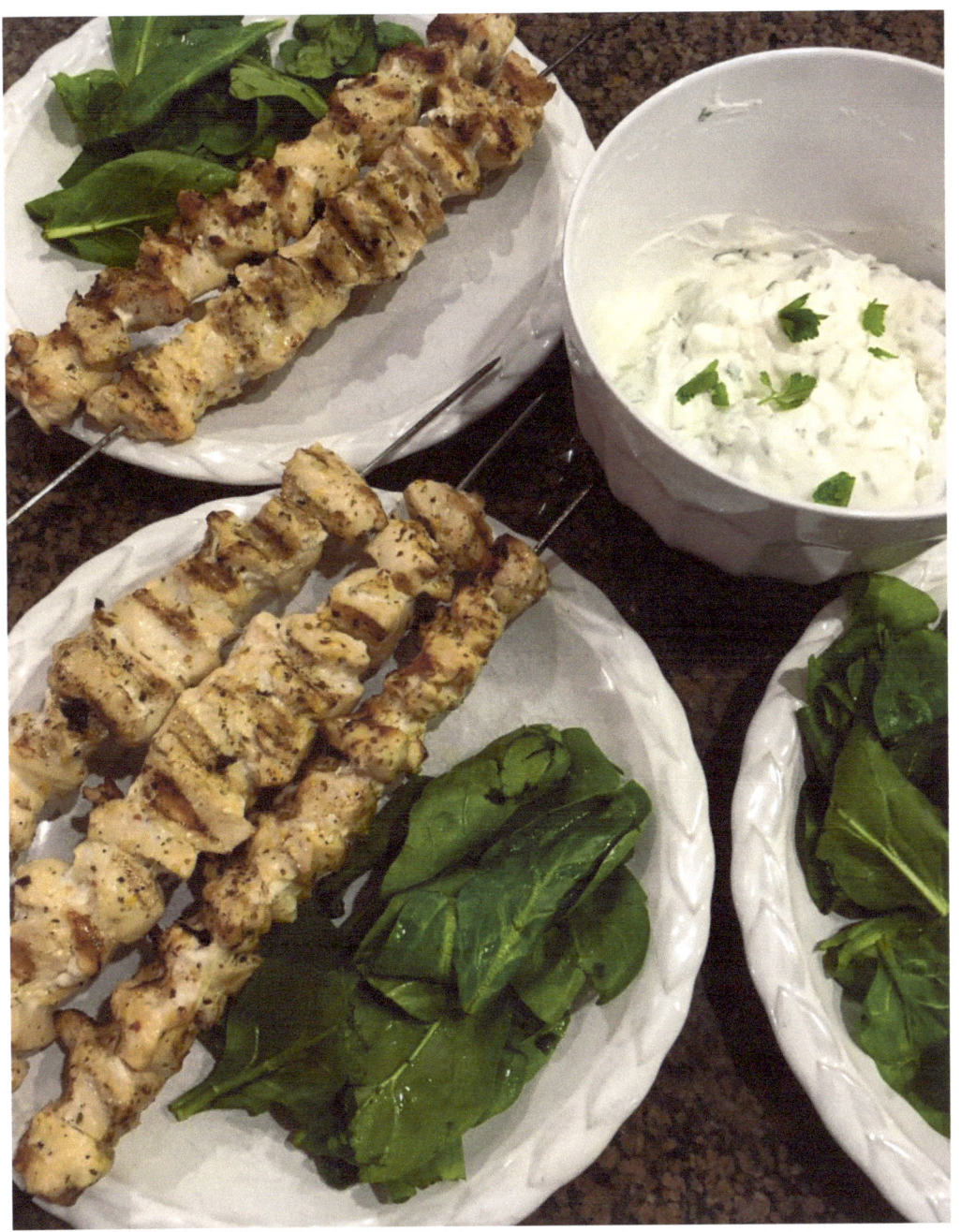

Ingredients:
4 large chicken breasts (approx. 3 ½ lbs)
2 tsp oregano
2 cloves garlic, minced
¼ cup olive oil (this can be reduced)
zest of 1 lemon
2 Tbsp fresh lemon juice
1 teaspoon red pepper flakes

Tzatziki Sauce:
2 cups plain Greek yogurt
1 cucumber
2 Tbsp parsley, chopped
2 Tbsp mint, chopped
1 Tbsp lemon juice
dash of Kosher salt and freshly ground pepper

Yield: 8 Kebabs + ½ cup Tzatziki Sauce

Directions:
1. Start the grill for medium-hot direct heat
2. Marinade: Combine olive oil, lemon juice, garlic, oregano, red pepper flakes and lemon zest.
3. Trim chicken breasts and cut into cubes. Add chicken to marinade and refrigerate for at least 30 minutes.
4. Meanwhile prepare the Tzatziki: Peel, seed and chop cucumber.
5. In a bowl, combine cucumber, yogurt, parsley, mint and
6. lemon juice. Season to taste with salt and pepper. Set aside, covered and refrigerate.
7. Thread chicken onto skewers, shaking off excess marinade. Grill chicken on both sides, turning as needed, until done, about 8 minutes.
8. Remove chicken from grill and serve with Tzatziki.

Calories: 263
Carbohydrates: 5g, Protein 43g, Fat 8g

Greek Marinated Pork Tenderloin

Ingredients:

(2) pork tenderloins (1 ½ lbs each)

¼ cup fresh lemon juice

¼ cup red wine vinegar

2 Tbsp olive oil

2 tsp minced fresh oregano

2 cloves garlic, minced

2 tsp Kosher salt

½ tsp ground pepper

Yield: (6) 5oz. Servings

Directions:

1. Whisk the vinegar, lemon juice, olive oil, garlic, oregano, salt and pepper together in a medium bowl. Pour into a 1-gallon lock-top bag, add the pork, and close the bag. Refrigerate for at least 1-2 hours.
2. Remove the pork from the marinade.
3. Heat grill on medium heat. Grill the tenderloins until the undersides are seared with grill marks about 2-5 minutes. Flip the pork tenderloins and continue grilling until temperature reads 155°F (slightly pink in the center).
4. Remove tenderloins from grill and let rest 10 minutes.
5. Slice tenderloins and serve!

Calories: 288
Carbohydrates: 3g, Protein 46g, Fat 10g

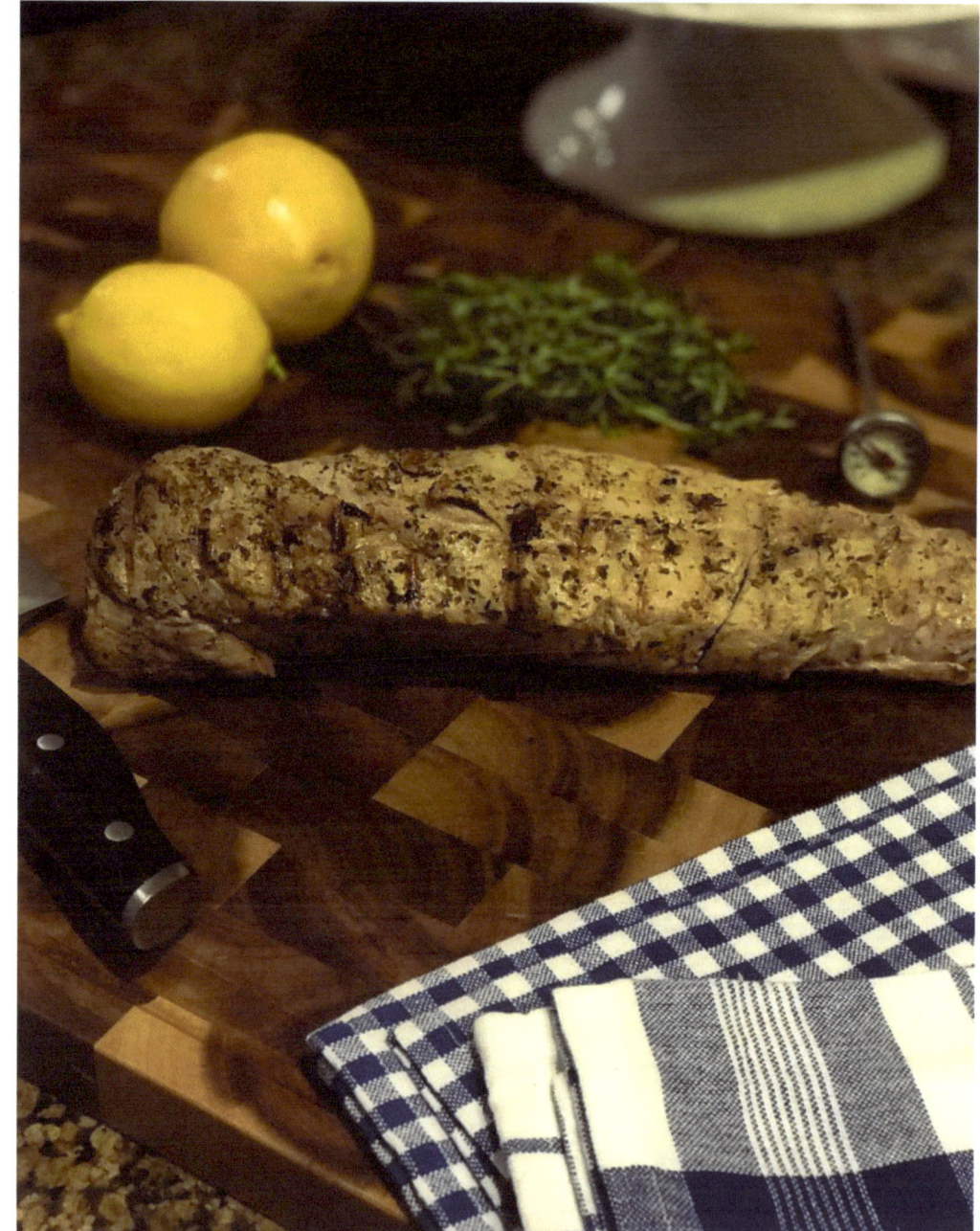

Latin Style Chicken and Black Bean Salad

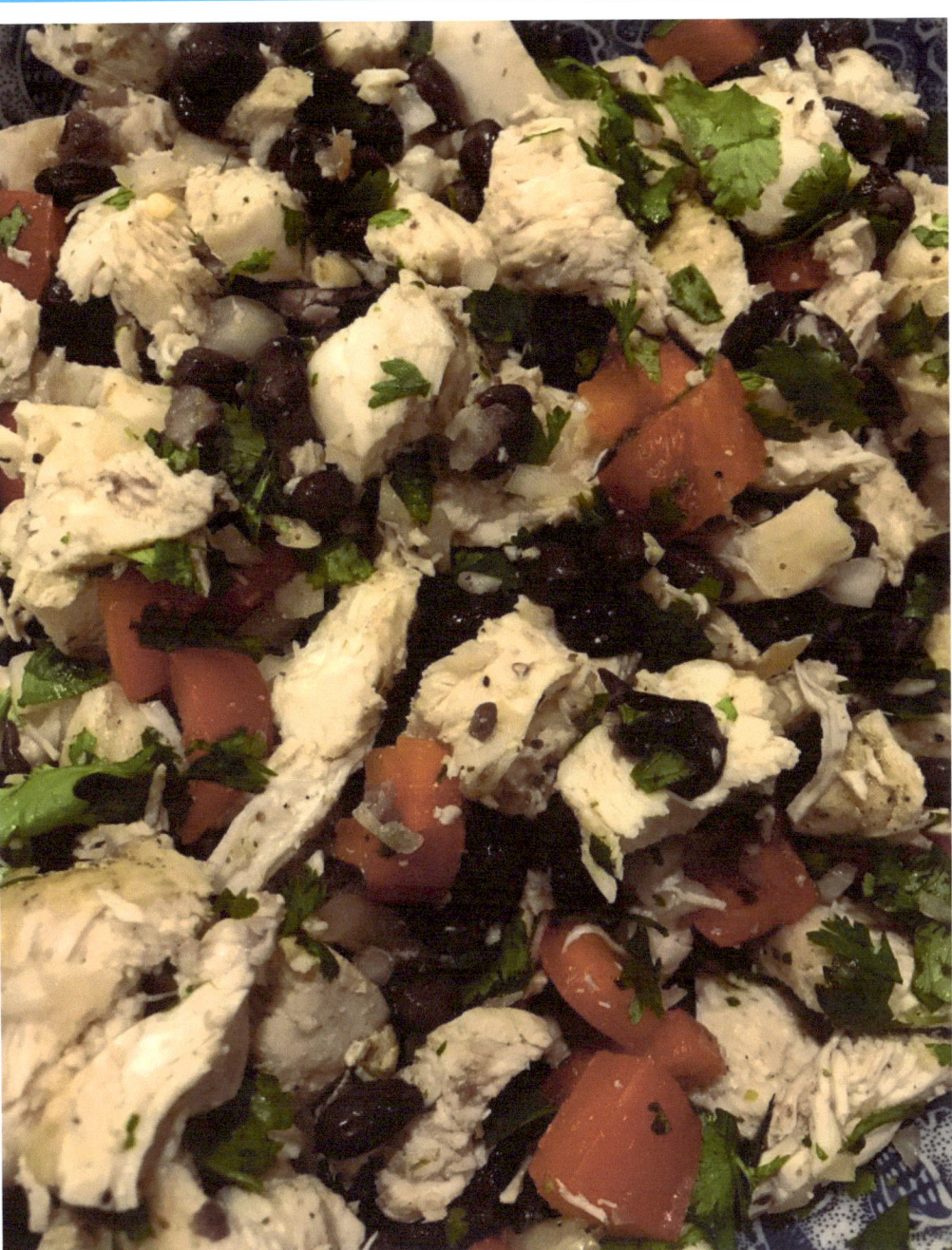

Ingredients:
2 cups baked or grilled chicken breast, cubed
(1) 15 oz. can of black beans, rinsed
1 large red bell pepper, chopped
¼ cup cilantro, chopped
4 cups salad greens

Serve with:
Cilantro Lime Jalapeño Dressing (see separate recipe)

Yield: 4 Servings

Directions:
1. Combine chicken, rinsed black beans, bell pepper, and ¼ cup cilantro in a medium bowl.
2. Divide chicken mixture into 4 servings.
3. Plate chicken mixture on top of 1 cup of greens.
4. Garnish with 2 Tbsp Cilantro Lime Jalapeño Dressing.

Calories: 242
Carbohydrates: 22g, Protein: 30g, Fat: 4g

Buffalo Chicken Casserole (recipe adapted from PaleOMG.com)

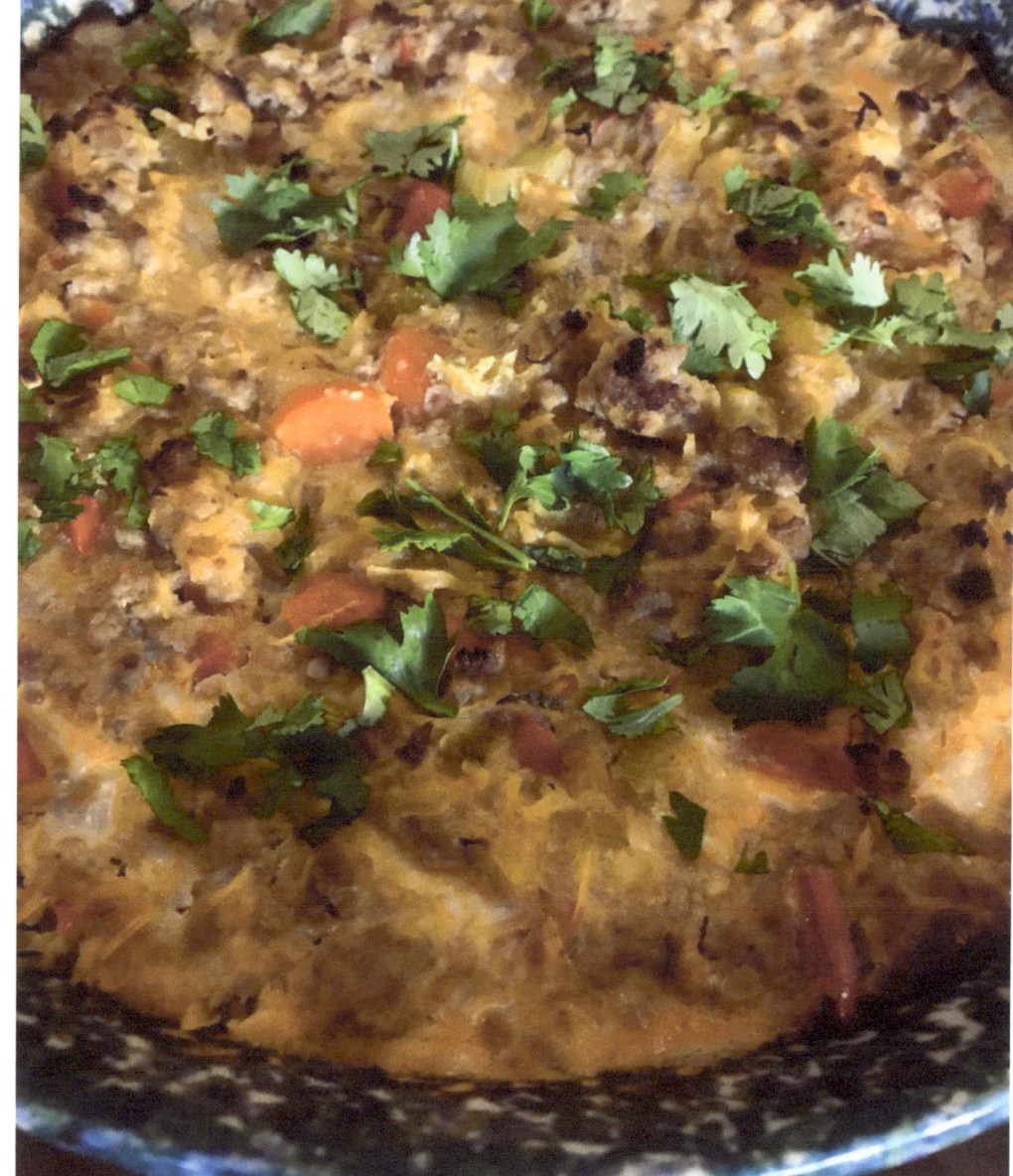

Ingredients:

- 2 cloves garlic
- 1 medium carrot
- 1 tsp garlic powder
- 1 tsp sea salt
- ¼ tsp ground pepper
- 6 oz. egg whites
- 2 lbs. 99% lean ground turkey
- ¼ cup olive oil Mayonaise
- 3 lb. spaghetti squash, cooked, seeded and strands separated
- 1 tsp olive oil
- 1 medium, red bell pepper
- 2 medium celery stalks
- ½ onion, chopped
- ½ cup Frank's hot sauce

Yield: 6 Servings

Directions:

1. Cook spaghetti squash as you would normally in oven or Instant Pot. Let cool. Remove seeds. Scrape squash from skin with fork to separate threads.
2. Spray large baking dish with non-stick spray and layer squash in the bottom of dish.
3. In a large pan over medium heat, heat olive oil. Add garlic, carrot, celery, onion, and bell pepper and cook for about 10 minutes, until the onion is translucent. Add the ground meat, salt, garlic powder and pepper and cook until the meat is no longer pink.
4. Remove from heat, and add hot sauce and mayo; mix well to combine. Add mixture to the baking dish and mix well with squash.
5. Add the whisked egg whites and mix everything together.
6. Bake for 1 hour or until the top forms a slight crust. Let rest for 5 minutes before serving.
7. Garnish with chopped scallion and avocado slices.

Calories: 290
Carbohydrates: 22g, Protein 40g, Fat 5.6g

Apricot Glazed Pork Tenderloin

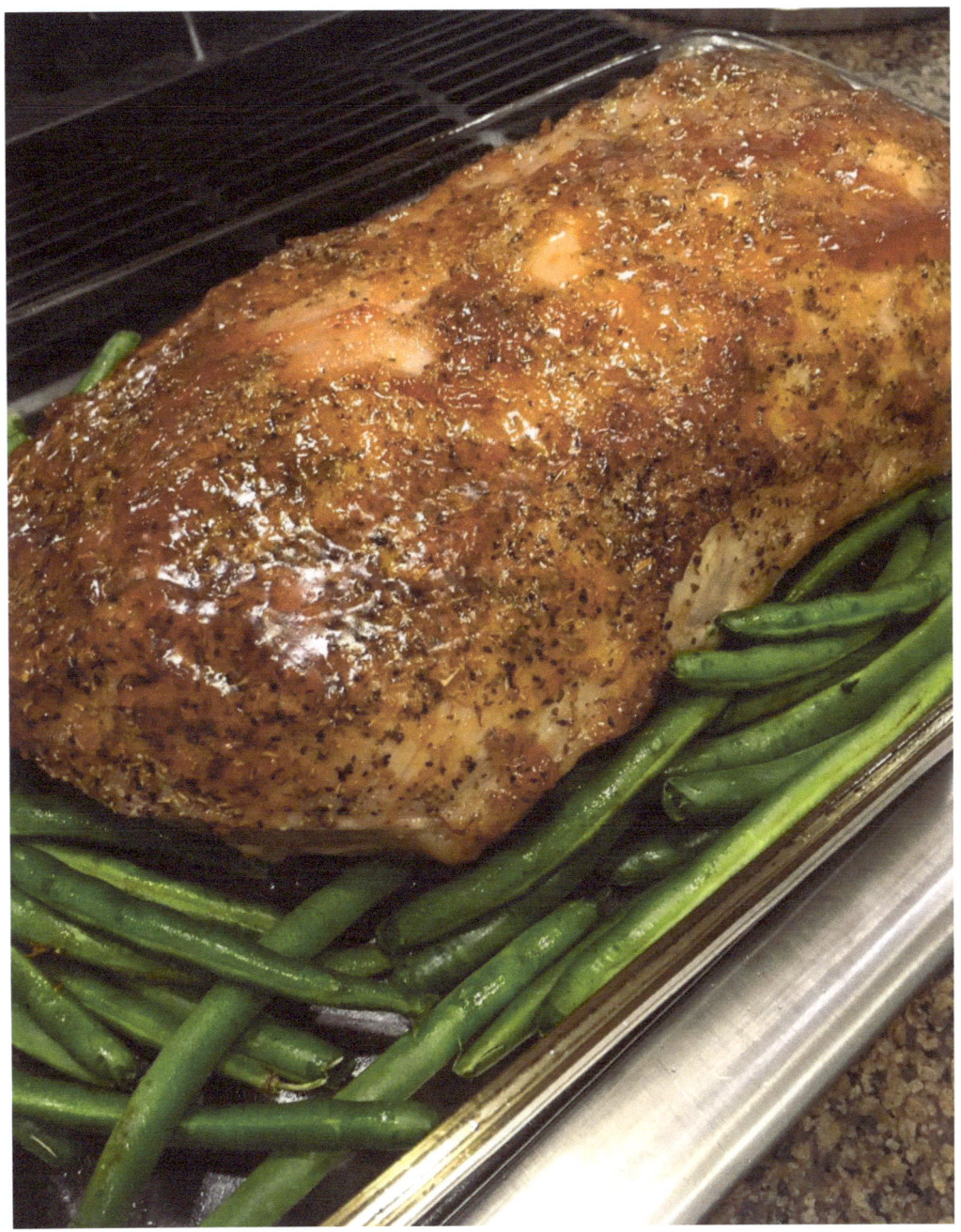

Ingredients:
1 (3lb or more) boneless pork loin, trimmed
½ cup apricot all fruit spread
1 teaspoon salt
1 teaspoon dried oregano
¾ teaspoon garlic powder
½ teaspoon freshly ground black pepper

Yield: 5lb tenderloin ~(14) 5oz. Servings

Directions:
1. Preheat oven to 425°F.
2. Place the preserves in a small saucepan over medium-low heat, and cook 10 minutes or until melted. Keep warm over low heat.
3. Combine salt, oregano, garlic powder, and pepper; rub evenly over pork. Place pork on a rack coated with cooking spray; place rack in a shallow roasting pan.
4. Bake at 425° for 30 minutes. Brush ¼ cup fruit spread evenly over pork. Bake an additional 10 minutes. Brush remaining preserves evenly over pork. Bake an additional 10 minutes or until thermometer registers 155° (slightly pink). Let stand 10 minutes before slicing.

Calories per 5 oz Serving: 268
Carbohydrates 21g, Protein: 37g,, Fat: 4g

Turkey Meatloaf Muffins (recipe adapted from bodybuilding.com)

Ingredients:
- 3 egg whites (3 oz.)
- 1 cup (39g dry) quick cooking oats
- 2 lbs (32 oz.) 99% lean ground turkey
- ½ cup onion, chopped
- 2 cloves garlic, minced
- 2 tsp dry yellow mustard
- ½ tsp ground cumin
- ½ tsp thyme
- 1 tsp salt
- 1 tsp ground black pepper
- 2 tsp lemon zest (optional)

Yield: 12 Muffins

Suggested Serving Size: 2-3

Directions:
1. Preheat oven to 375°F
2. Spray muffin pan/silicon mold with olive oil spritzer or cooking spray.
3. Add oats to egg whites; let stand 5 minutes.
4. In large bowl, add all ingredients and mix well.
5. Using a 1/3 measuring cup, scoop out turkey mixture and form into balls and place into muffin pan.
6. Bake for 40 minutes.
7. Set oven to broil and cook meatballs a few more minutes until tops are browned.

Calories per muffin: 124
Carbohydrates: 6g, Protein 21g, Fat 1g

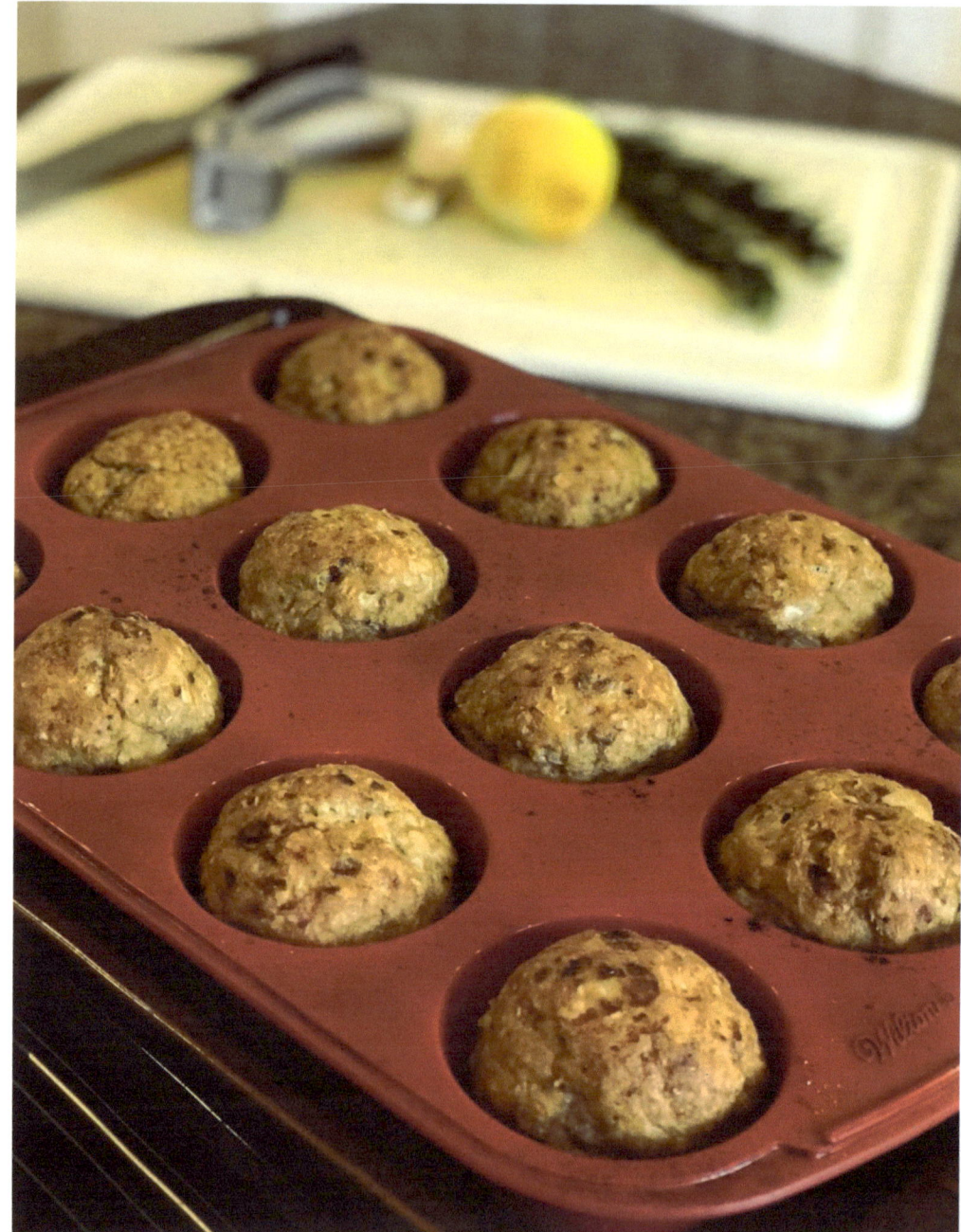

Grilled Salmon with Orange Ginger Mustard Glaze

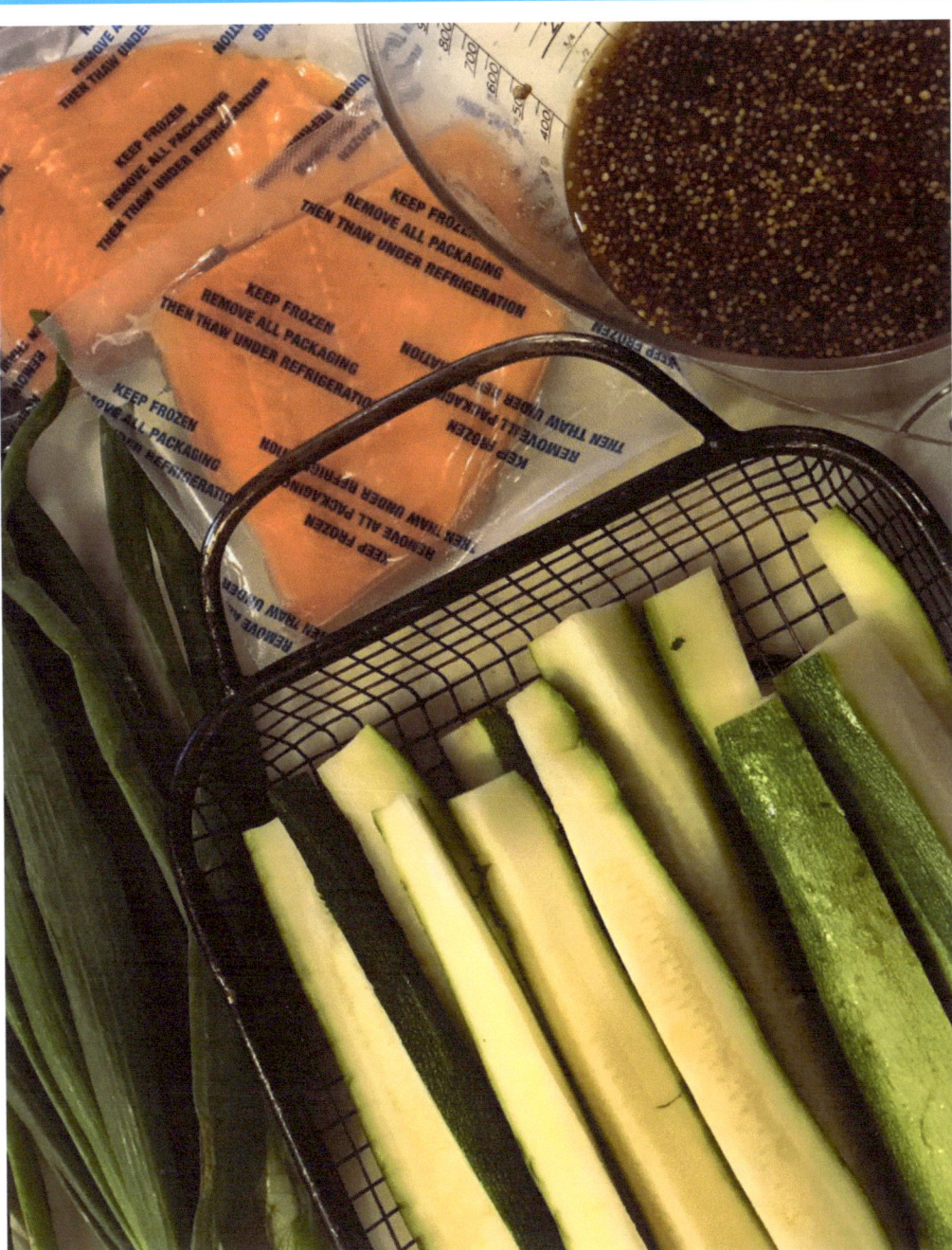

Ingredients:
4 (6-ounce) Salmon fillets
2 Tbsp fresh grated ginger
2 Tbsp honey

Marinade/Glaze:
¼ cup fresh orange juice
¼ cup tamari or low-sodium soy sauce
¼ cup Dijon Mustard
¼ cup cream sherry (optional)

Yield: 1 cup Glaze/Marinade

Serving Size: (4) 6 oz. Salmon Filets with 1-2 Tbsp Glaze

Directions:
1. Combine glaze ingredients in a small bowl and mix thoroughly.
2. Transfer glaze to a zip-lock bag. Add fish to bag; seal and marinate in refrigerator 30 for at least 30 minutes.
3. Remove fish from bag; reserve marinade.
4. Preheat grill to medium-high heat.
5. Transfer salmon to prepared grill and cook until done (about 5 minutes/side) or until fish flakes easily when tested with a fork.
6. Place remaining marinade in a saucepan; bring to a boil. Serve with fish: garnish with green onions and lemon slices if desired.

Glaze/Marinade Calories per Tbsp: 29
Carbohydrates: 3g, Protein 1g, Fat 1g

Shrimp and Scallop Stir Fry

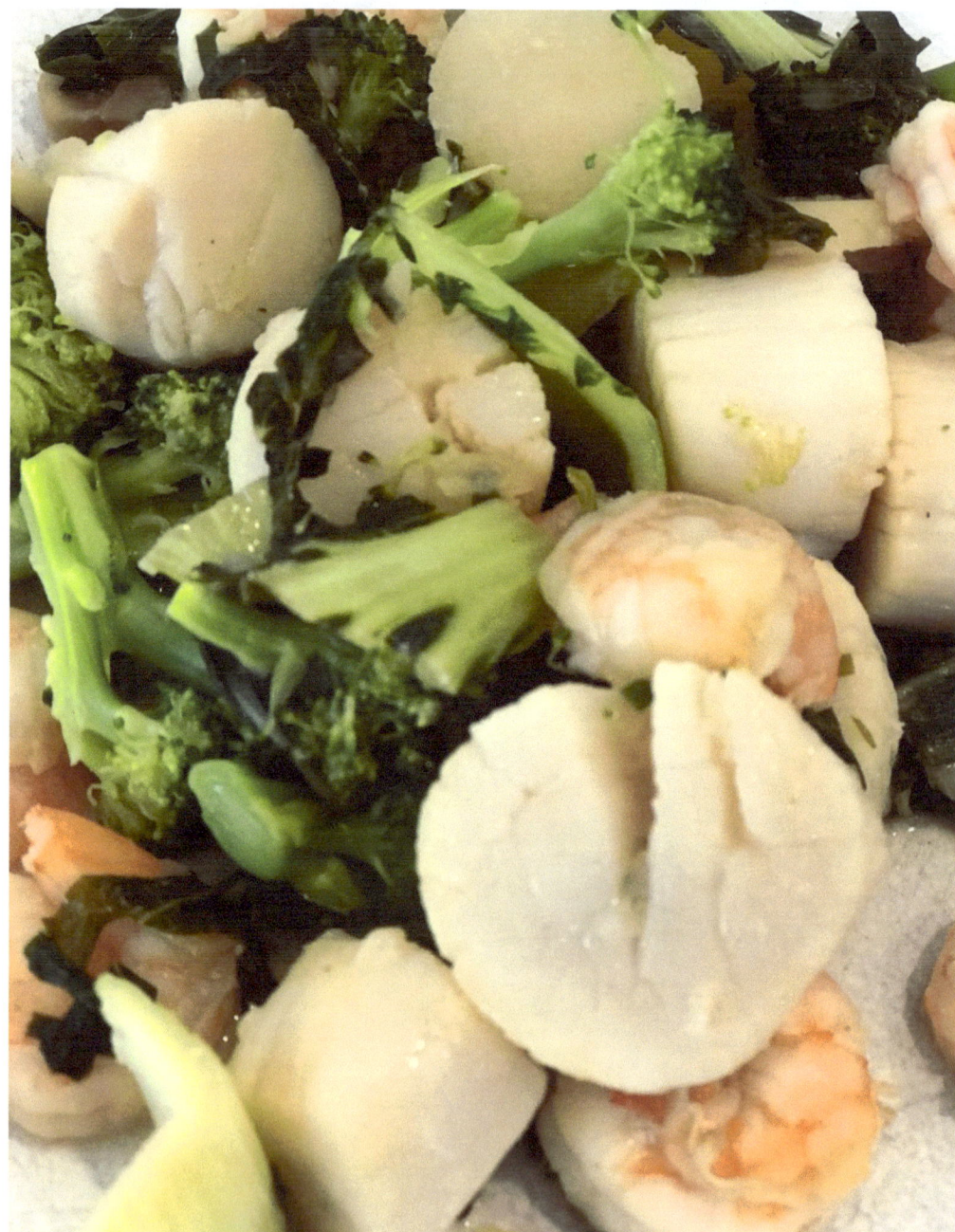

Ingredients:
- ¾ lb shrimp
- ¾ lb scallops
- ½ Tbsp Sesame Oil
- 1 Tbsp low-sodium Soy Sauce
- 2 Tbsp green onions, chopped
- 1 Tbsp zested ginger
- 1 Tbsp fresh lemon juice
- 1 tsp Sriracha
- 1 cup snow peas
- 1 cup mushrooms, sliced
- ½ cup onion, chopped
- 1 cup water chestnuts (drained)
- 2 cups baby Bok choy, chopped
- 1 Tbsp extra virgin olive oil
- 1 clove garlic

Yield: 4 Servings

Directions:
1. Heat 1 Tbsp extra virgin olive oil in wok or large pan.
2. Cook vegetables until soft (approximately 10 minutes).
3. Add seafood and all other ingredients.
4. Cook an additional 6 minutes or until shrimp and scallops are fully cooked.

Calories: 232
Carbohydrates: 15g, Protein 25g, Fat 8g

Crab Cakes

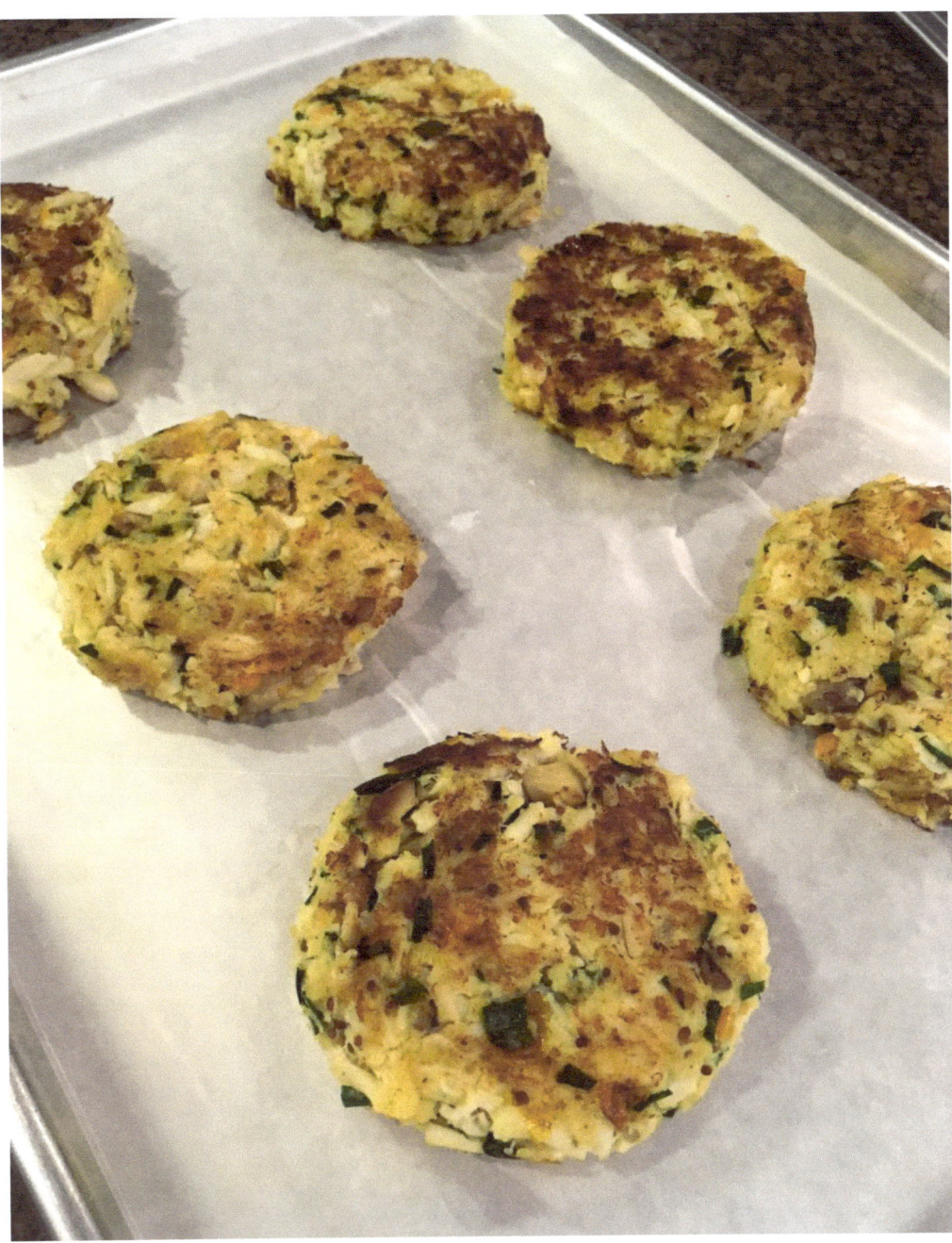

Ingredients:
½ cup diced scallions
2 egg whites (¼ cup)
2 tsp Old Bay seasoning
3 Tbsp olive oil mayo
½ tsp baking powder
½ cup baby Portabello mushrooms, finely chopped
½ cup red bell pepper, finely chopped
1 tsp horseradish
8 drops Sriracha sauce
½ cup panko
2 tsp fresh lemon juice
1 lb. lump crab meat
pinch of salt and pepper

Yield: 6 Crab Cakes

Directions:
1. Whip together first 5 ingredients and chill.
2. Sauté mushrooms and bell pepper with 2 tsp extra virgin olive oil and a pinch of salt and pepper. Set aside and let cool.
3. Once cooled, add both mixtures together.
4. In a separate bowl, combine the horseradish and next 5 ingredients. Fold everything together and form into 6 crab cakes.
5. Sear each side in pan with extra virgin olive oil.
6. Bake in oven at 375°F for 6-8 minutes.
7. Enjoy!

Calories per Crab Cake: 120
Carbohydrates: 8g, Protein 20g, Fat 2g

Spicy Tuna Poke Bowls

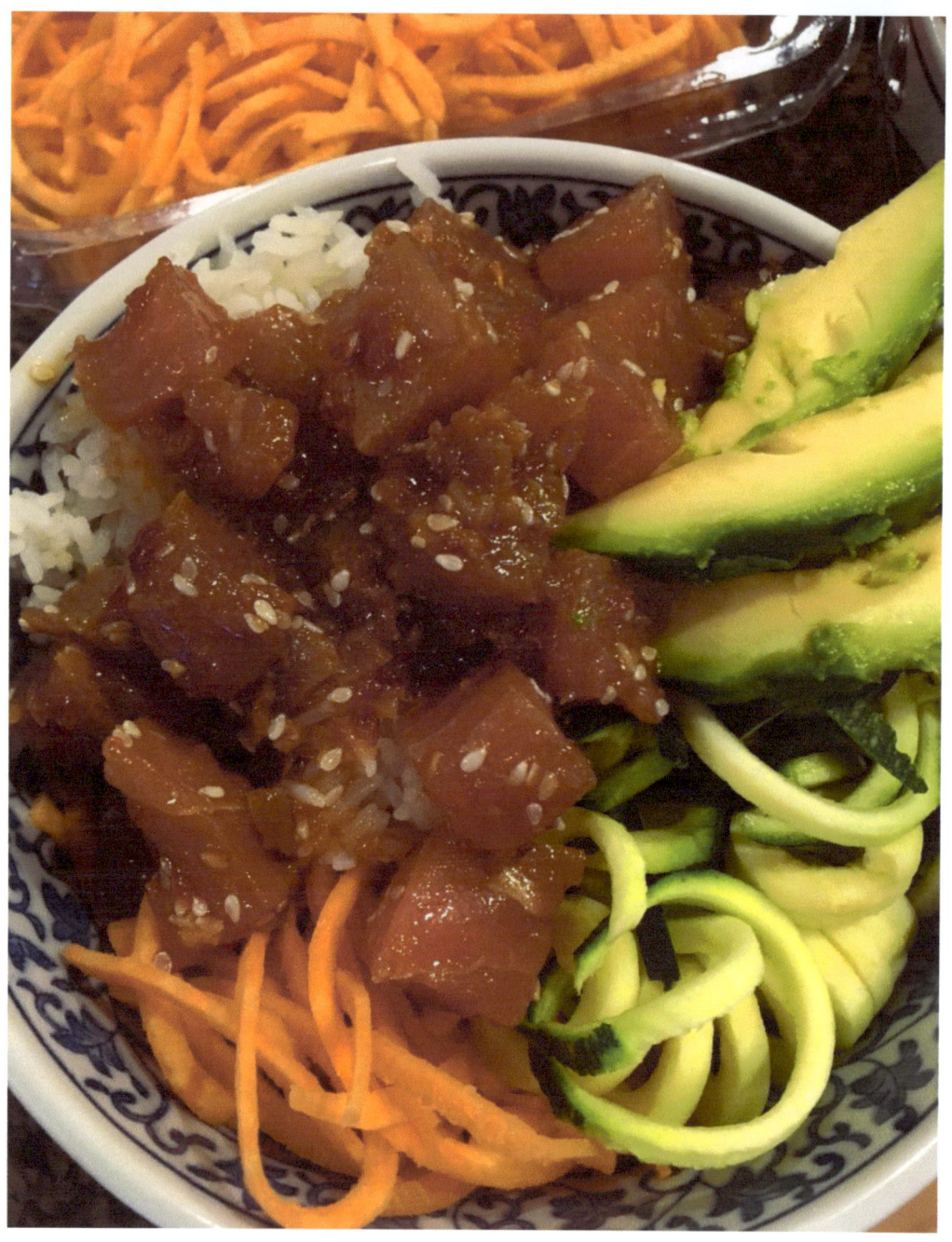

Ingredients:

Spicy Tuna:
1.5 lbs sashimi-grade tuna, cubed
¼ cup Bragg's liquid aminos
2 Tbsp Sambal Oelek (Thai chili paste)
2 Tbsp fresh ginger, minced
1 Tbsp rice vinegar
1 Tbsp toasted sesame oil
1 Tbsp toasted sesame seeds

Spicy Mayo:
¼ cup olive oil mayonnaise
2 Tbsp Sriracha
½ tsp toasted sesame oil
2-3 drops fish sauce

Serve with:
cilantro, brown rice, avocado, seaweed salad, pickled ginger, zoodles, cucumbers, green onions

Yield: 5 Servings

Directions:
1. Combine the liquid aminos, Sambal Oelek, ginger, rice vinegar, sesame oil and seeds and whisk until well incorporated. Add the cubed tuna to the bowl and stir gently to coat. Refrigerate for at least 20-30 minutes.
2. Meanwhile prepare rice as directed.
3. Prepare and slice toppings such as avocado, veggie spirals, seaweed salad, cucumber slices, etc.
4. Prepare spicy mayo (if desired) by combining all 4 ingredients until well mixed.
5. To serve: place ½ cup of rice at the bottom of each bowl, top with your choice of vegetables and then spoon the tuna over the veggies, dividing it equally between 5 bowls.

Calories: 226 (Spicy Tuna Only)
Carbohydrates: 2g, Protein 34g, Fat 3g

Coconut Peanut Butter Protein Balls

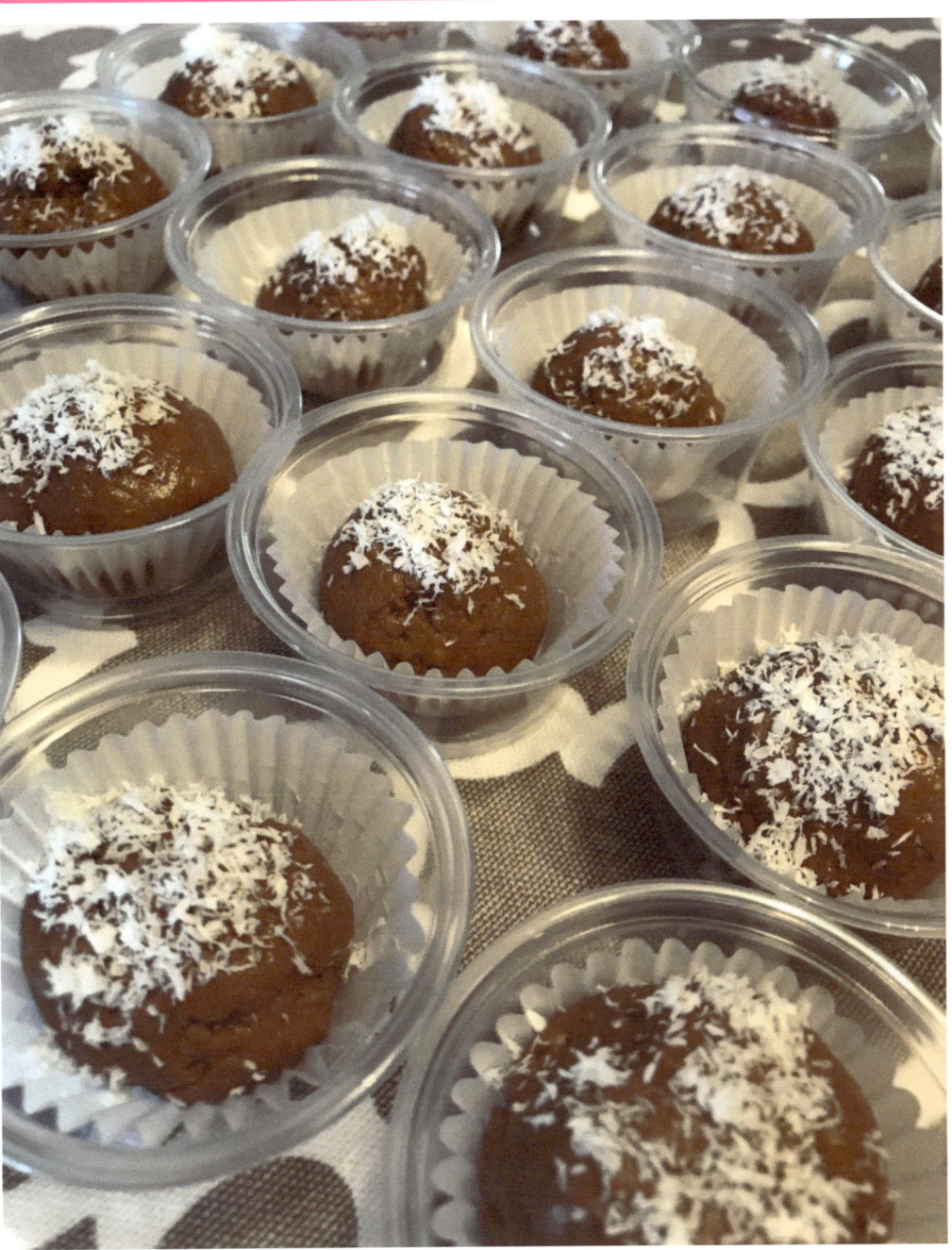

Ingredients:
1 cup creamy natural peanut butter
½ cup unsweetened coconut
½ cup honey
1-2 scoops chocolate protein powder

Toppings: (optional, not included in macros)
unsweetened coconut
crushed pretzels
crushed almonds

Yield: 24 Servings

Directions:
1. In a large bowl, combine peanut butter, honey and coconut.
2. Add 1 scoop protein powder and mix thoroughly.
3. Continue to add protein powder ¼ scoop at a time and mix until dough is not sticky.
4. Use a scoop to form 1" balls.
5. Line condiment containers with mini cupcake liners.
6. Place protein balls in lined containers.
7. Garnish with your favorite topping.
8. These treats freeze well!
9. Macros will vary depending on the protein powder you use!

Calories per serving: 101
Carbohydrates 9g, Protein 3g, Fat 7g

Energy Balls

Ingredients:
½ cup creamy natural peanut butter
¼ cup dried cherries
½ cup nuts, crushed
¼ cup s/f mini chocolate chips
1 Tbsp chia seeds
¼ cup unsweetened coconut
2 Tbsp honey
1 cup Quaker Oats
Pinch of sea salt (optional)

Yield: 20 Servings

Directions:
1. In a large bowl, combine all ingredients.
2. Use a scoop to form 1" balls.
3. Press and roll firmly to make into ball shape.
4. These treats freeze well!

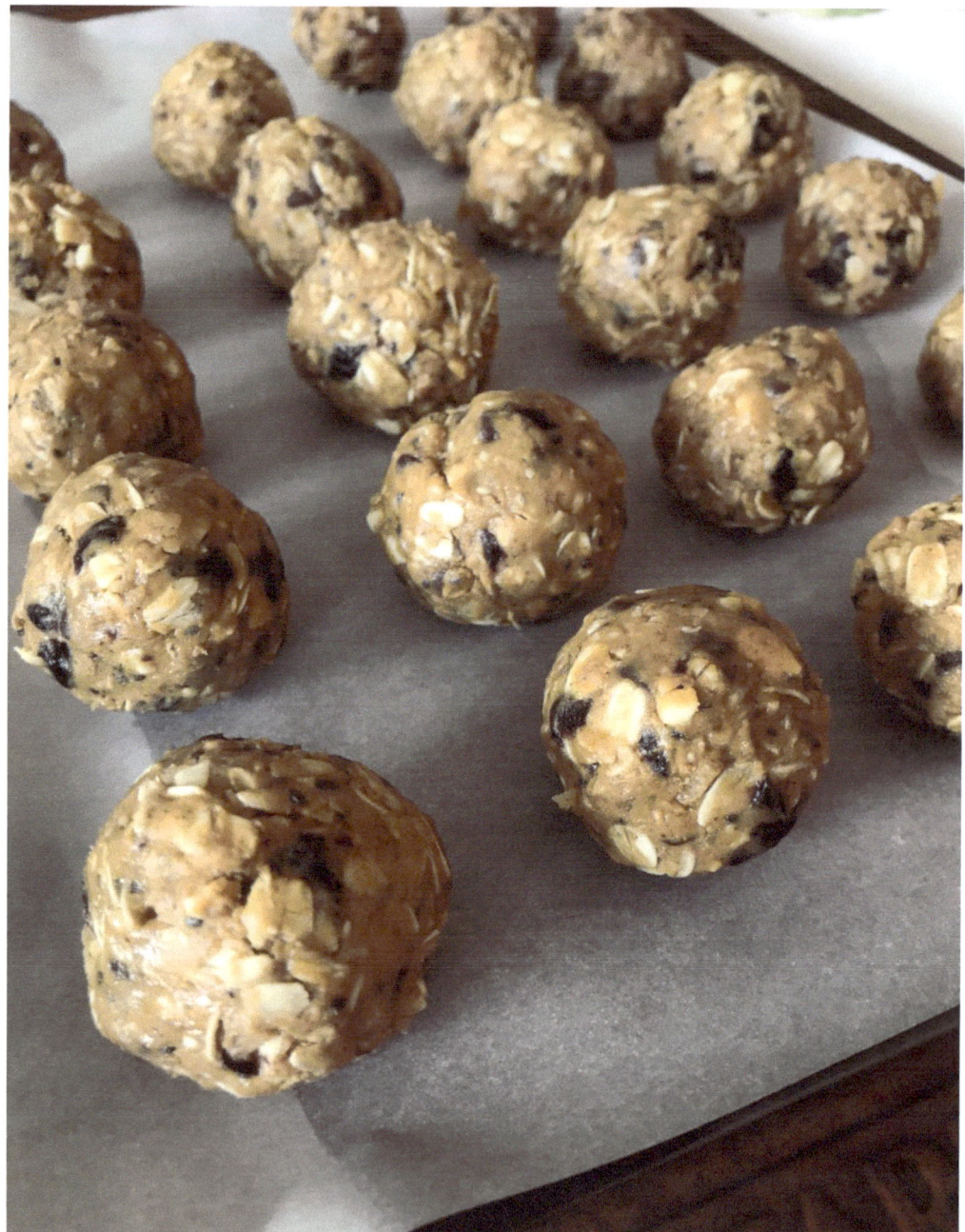

Calories per Energy Ball: 109
Carbohydrates: 9.5g, Protein: 3.3g, Fat: 7g

Black Cherry Protein Smoothie Bowl

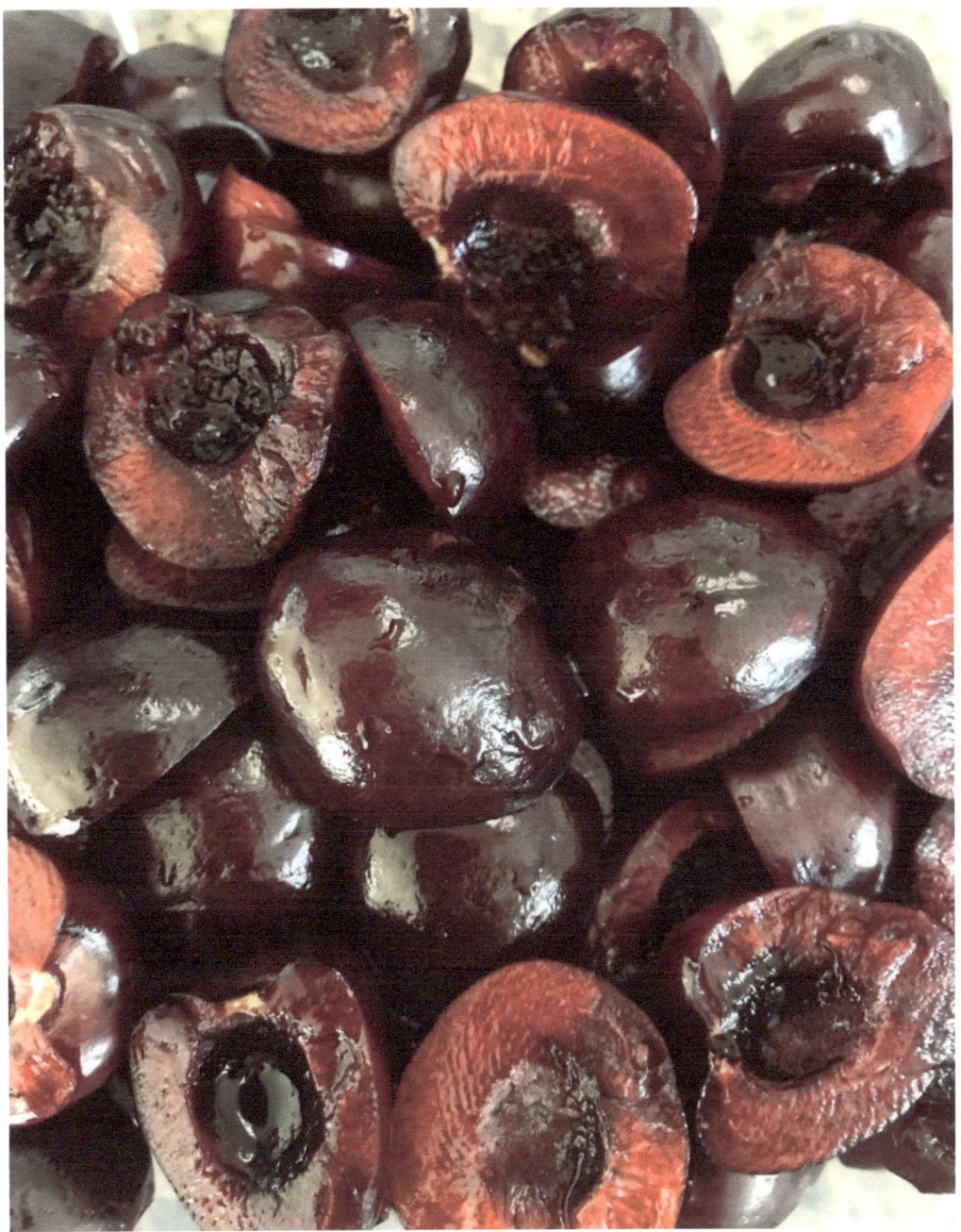

Ingredients:
2 cups pitted black cherries
2 frozen bananas
1 cup unsweetened almond milk
2 Tbsp almond butter
1 scoop vanilla protein powder

Toppings:
(optional; not included in macros)
Unsweetened Coconut
Crushed almonds
Granola
Sliced banana

Yield: 4 Servings

Directions:
1. Remove pits from cherries and freeze.
2. Place all ingredients in a blender.
3. Puree until smooth.
4. Divide between 4 bowls.
5. Macros will vary depending on the protein powder you use!

Calories per serving: 230
Carbohydrates: 30.4g, Protein 7.5g, Fat 10.5g

Lemon Chickpea Muffins

Ingredients:
- 1 ¾ cup Chickpeas (15 oz. can)
- zest from two lemons (2 tsp)
- zest from one orange (1 tsp)
- 2 Tbsp fresh lemon juice
- 2 Tbsp orange juice
- ¼ cup extra-virgin olive oil
- ¼-½ cup Stevia (to taste)
- 2 egg yolks
- 2/3 cup whole-wheat flour
- 2 tsp baking powder
- ½ tsp salt
- ½ tsp ground cardamom
- ½ cup almond flour
- 2 egg whites

Yield: 24 Mini Muffins

Serving Size: 1-2 Muffins

Directions:
1. Preheat oven to 325°F.
2. Spray Muffin tin lightly with olive oil mister.
3. Puree chickpeas in food processor or blender until smooth. Add zest and juice from lemon and oranges, olive oil, stevia and egg yolks. Blend until smooth.
4. Sift together flour, almond flour, baking powder, salt and cardamom. Stir in chickpea mixture. Whisk egg whites until they hold semisoft peaks. Fold egg whites into batter.
5. Scoop batter into muffin tin.
6. In small bowl, combine ground almonds, sugar and cardamom. Set aside for topping.
7. Sprinkle topping mixture onto each muffin (optional)
8. Bake 12-13 minutes, or until toothpick inserted into center comes out clean.

Calories per muffin : 61
Carbohydrates: 9.8g, Protein 2.2g, Fat: 3.7g

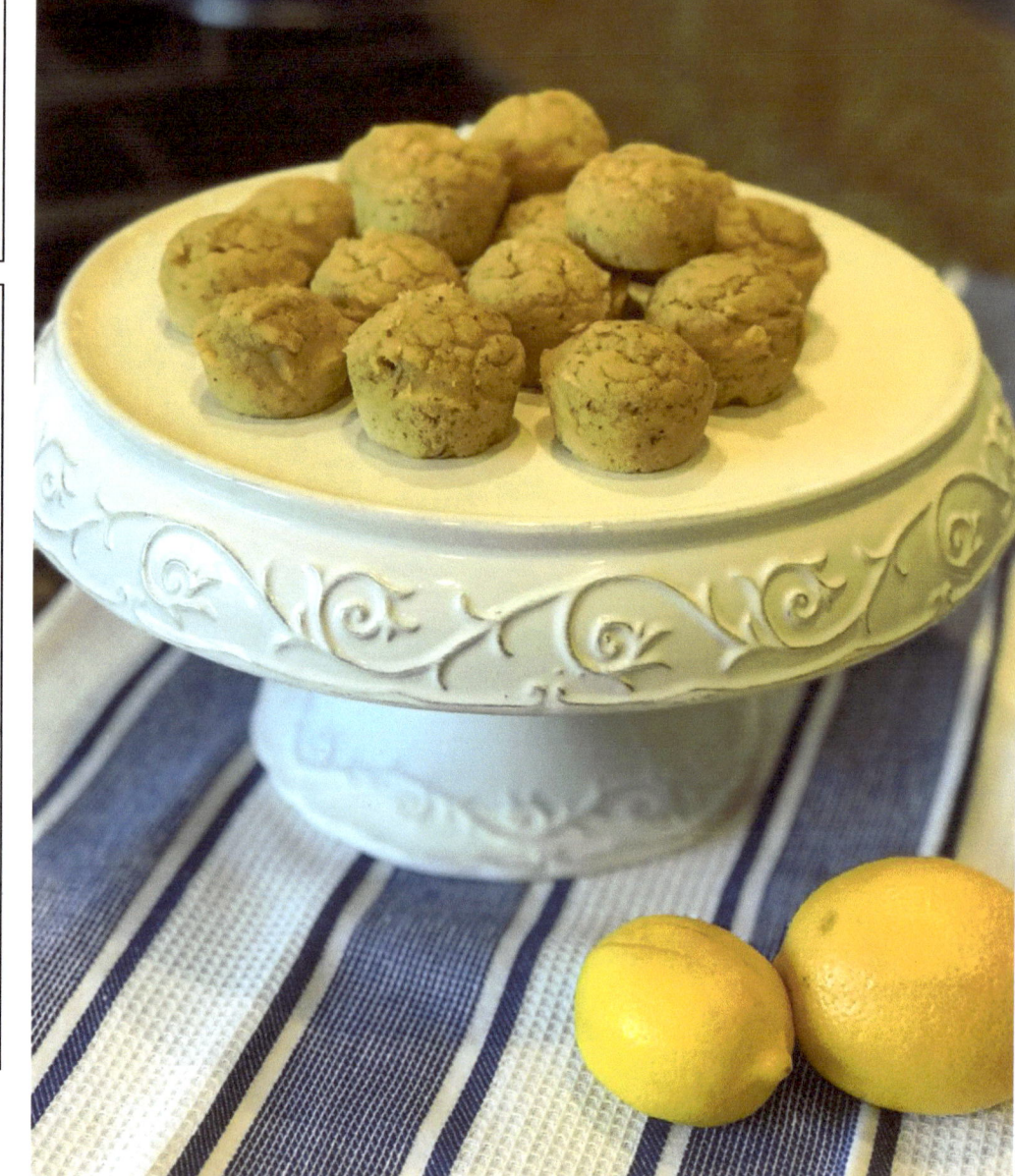

At KK Wellness Consulting

...we educate, inspire, and empower our clients to lead healthy lifestyles using a cognitive behavioral approach coupled with whole food nutrition. We teach our clients how to eat clean and how to fuel their bodies. Our Facebook KK Wellness subscription page keeps our clients connected with a sense of community and is loaded with rich content: recipes, cooking demonstrations, product reviews, workouts, and more…. everything you need to support your healthy lifestyle journey.

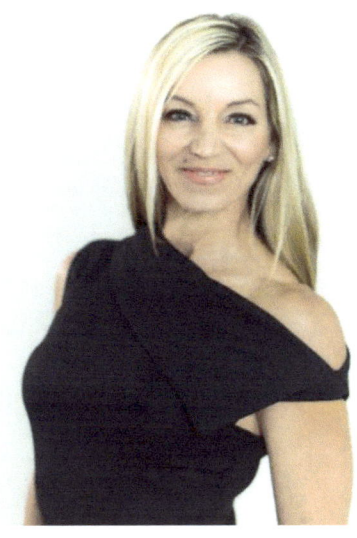

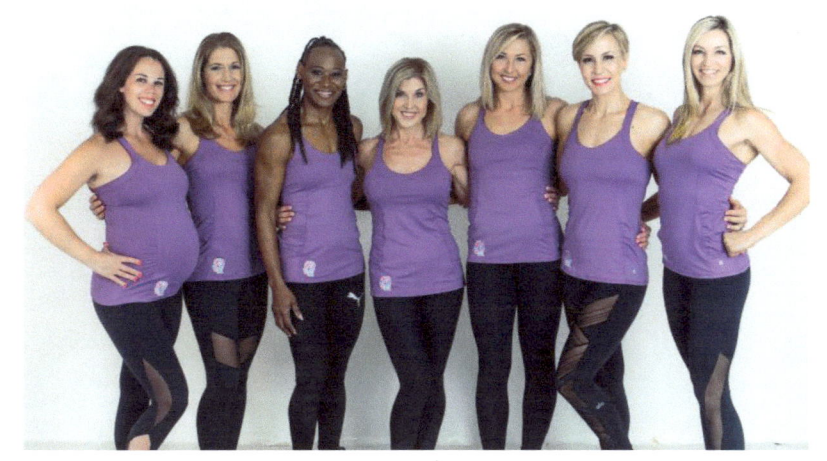

Brandy Flotten is one of the behavioral nutrition coaches at KKW. In addition to coaching, her role at KKW is to create recipes, perform cooking demonstrations, and hold on-line workshops. She is passionate about the power of nutrition and loves to teach people how to feed their families.

Kelly Killen (pictured in center) is a licensed behavior analyst with the Virginia Medical Board, and the founder and lead coach of KK Wellness. Her diversified team of licensed and certified coaches offers services in nutrition coaching, custom meal plans, custom workouts and more.

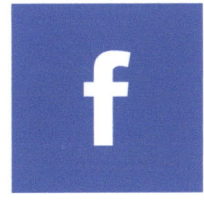

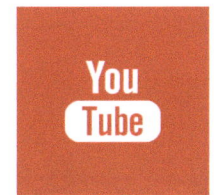
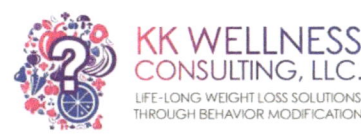

KK WELLNESS CONSULTING, LLC.
LIFE-LONG WEIGHT LOSS SOLUTIONS THROUGH BEHAVIOR MODIFICATION

Search for us on social media; our tagline is:

#preppingforlife

www.ingramcontent.com/pod-product-compliance
Lightning Source LLC
Chambersburg PA
CBHW041324290426

44108CB00005B/125